DATE DUE

 SAGE Publications
International Educational and Professional Publisher
Thousand Oaks   London   New Delhi

For information:

SAGE Publications, Inc.
2455 Teller Road
Thousand Oaks, California 91320
E-mail: order@sagepub.com

SAGE Publications Ltd.
6 Bonhill Street
London EC2A 4PU
United Kingdom

SAGE Publications India Pvt. Ltd.
M-32 Market
Greater Kailash I
New Delhi 110 048 India

Printed in the United States of America

Library of Congress Cataloging-in-Publication Data

Knapp, Thomas R., 1930–
Quantitative nursing research / by Thomas R. Knapp.
p. cm.
Includes bibliographical references (p.   ) and index.
ISBN 0-7619-1362-9 (cloth : acid-free paper).—
ISBN 0-7619-1363-7 (pbk.: acid-free paper)
1. Nursing—Research—Methodology. 2. Nursing—Research–Statistical methods.
I. Title.
RT81.5.K59 1998
610.73'07'27—dc21   97-45338

This book is printed on acid-free paper.

99 98 00 01 02 03 10 9 8 7 6 5 4 3 2 1

Acquiring Editor:	Dan Ruth
Editorial Assitant:	Anna Howland
Production Editor:	Sanford Robinson
Editorial Assistant:	Denise Santoyo
Designer/Typesetter:	Rose Tylak
Cover Designer:	Kristi White
Print Buyer:	Anna Chin

Contents

Preface

I am not a nurse. But I am a nursing researcher, having contributed to the research literature in nursing, served as a reviewer for nursing research journals, and co-authored a dictionary of nursing theory and research. I have held joint appointments in nursing and education for approximately 20 years, first at the University of Rochester and presently at The Ohio State University.

This book is intended to serve as a textbook for master's and doctoral students in nursing and as a reference source for nursing researchers. The content is restricted to quantitative research methods. The word "quantitative" is a cover term for those methods that traditionally are associated with research in the physical sciences and several of the social sciences, most notably experiments, surveys, and correlational studies of various types. This is not meant to imply that quantitative methods are in any way superior to qualitative methods in nursing research. The word "qualitative" is itself a cover term for those methods that traditionally are associated with research in the humanities and other social sciences, namely ethnography, grounded theory, phenomenology, and related approaches to the advancement of knowledge. The absence of attention to qualitative methods is merely an acknowledgment of my limited expertise. If you would like to study qualitative methods, then I refer you to the specialized qualitative research texts and to those portions of general nursing research texts that deal with qualitative approaches.

I have divided the text into five main parts of four chapters each. The first part (Chapters 1-4) deals with research in general and quantitative nursing research in particular, concentrating on matters such as what research is; how to formulate research questions and hypotheses; issues of causality, generalizability, and randomization; and ethical considerations in nursing research. The second part covers research design and consists of a chapter on experiments (Chapter 5), a chapter on surveys (Chapter 6), and two chapters on correlational research (Chapters 7 and 8). I estimate that those three types of designs are used, singly or in combination with one another, in approximately 90% of quantitative nursing research studies and approximately 70% of all nursing research studies.

The third part is devoted to matters of sampling (Chapter 9), measurement (Chapter 10), statistics (Chapter 11), and the use of computers (Chapter 12). The emphasis in that part of the book, as in all other parts, is on concepts, not formulas or equations (none are provided). The fourth part addresses some specialized approaches to nursing research. Chapter 13 treats secondary analysis, Chapter 14 is on meta-analysis, Chapter 15 discusses both pilot studies and replication studies, and Chapter 16 deals with methodological research.

The final part is concerned with studying subjects one at a time (Chapter 17), the measurement of change (Chapter 18), missing-data problems (Chapter 19), and research dissemination (Chapter 20). A list of references and an index complete the work. References that are relevant to a particular chapter also are provided at the end of that chapter.

For examples, I have drawn heavily from *Nursing Research* and *Research in Nursing & Health,* two of the peer-reviewed nursing research journals that are highly regarded and publish large numbers of quantitative research reports. (Both also publish the reports of qualitative studies.) I also refer frequently to the Physicians' Health Study and the Nurses' Health Study. Although both of those studies satisfy only a broad definition of nursing research, the former is a classic example of an experiment and the latter is a classic example of a survey, two of the quantitative research methods that are emphasized in this book.

At the end of each chapter, there are one or more study suggestions that are designed to help reinforce the material contained in the chapter. Most of these involve reading and critiquing—positively and negatively—quantitative nursing research articles.

A word about definitions: Most, if not all, of the definitions used in this book have been excerpted in whole or in part from *A Dictionary of Nursing Theory and Research* (2nd ed., Sage, 1995), co-authored by Bethel A. Powers and myself, to which reference already has been made. You should consult that source if you need further clarification of particular terms.

I thank Jean Brown and Nancy Campbell-Heider of the State University of New York at Buffalo, Teresa Julian of Otterbein College, Laura

Kimble of Emory University, Bethel Powers of the University of Rochester, and my colleagues and students in the College of Nursing and College of Education at The Ohio State University (especially Jennie Nickel) for the help they have given me, directly and indirectly, in the preparation of this book. I hasten to add that I relieve them of any errors of commission or omission that may remain. Those are all mine.

Thomas R. Knapp
The Ohio State University

To Jean and Laura

PART A

THE FOUNDATIONS OF QUANTITATIVE NURSING RESEARCH

The four chapters in the first part of this book all are relatively short, but they provide the necessary background for quantitative nursing research in general.

Chapter 1 contains a discussion of several basic terms (*research, theory, science*, etc.) and includes citations to some prototypical quantitative nursing research studies.

Chapter 2 deals with the usual starting points of scientific investigations—research questions and hypotheses, how they should be stated, how they differ from one another, and the like. This chapter also refers to several "live" nursing research examples to illustrate the phrasing of research questions, hypotheses, and purposes.

Chapter 3 is my favorite chapter. Nothing is more difficult and more challenging than the pursuit of causality and generalizability and understanding the role that randomization plays in both pursuits. You should pay particular attention to the section on random assignment versus random sampling. People always are getting them mixed up.

Chapter 4, the final chapter in this part, is concerned with research ethics with respect to both people (human subjects) and animals (infrahuman subjects). Most of nursing research involves people, but an important small percentage of quantitative nursing research studies consists of basic research on animals with ultimate implications for the health care of humans. You also should pay attention to the distinction between anonymity and confidentiality. People always are getting them mixed up too!

CHAPTER 1

What Is Quantitative Nursing Research?

CHAPTER OUTLINE

What Is Research?
What Sorts of Things "Count" as Research, and What Sorts of Things Do Not?
What Is Nursing?
What Do We Mean by "Quantitative"?
Therefore, What Is Quantitative Nursing Research?
Purposes of Nursing Research
Data-Gathering Techniques
What Is Science?
Study Suggestion

Key Terms: research, theory, basic research, applied research, data, science

WHAT IS RESEARCH?

Most definitions of **research** have at least two elements in common:

1. Research usually involves a careful and systematic investigation of some phenomenon.
2. The purpose of most research is to contribute to the advancement of knowledge.

Thus, research is an investigative activity that has as its goal the advancement of knowledge.

WHAT SORTS OF THINGS "COUNT" AS RESEARCH, AND WHAT SORTS OF THINGS DO NOT?

That is not an easy question to answer, but the following guidelines may be helpful in identifying activities that are *not* research:

1. If an activity consists of conjectures regarding the underlying reasons for particular results, then it should not be called research. That is the province of *theory*.
2. If an activity involves a *search* for available information (e.g., investigating the capabilities of different computer systems and searching for best value for money spent), then it is not research.
3. If an activity is concerned primarily with the organization or reorganization of knowledge, then it also should not be called research. The prototypical example of such an activity is a critique of books and articles that results in a synthesized written report (a literature review) or the writing of a textbook such as this one. Most authors of these types of materials, including myself in this particular endeavor, usually do not *add* to or advance knowledge; they simply redistribute it.
4. If an activity has a heavy polemic emphasis, then it is not research. Books and articles that express strong opinions, particularly those that do not provide any evidence in support of such opinions, are examples of nonresearch.

In this book, I provide a variety of examples of activities that *are* research. Most have in common the two criteria included in the preceding definition, namely, the careful and systematic investigation of some phenomenon and the addition to general knowledge.

WHAT IS NURSING?

I adopt the American Nurses Association's (ANA) definition of nursing as "the diagnosis and treatment of human responses to actual or potential health problems" (ANA, 1980, p. 9) and its later reiteration and elaboration (ANA, 1995, pp. 5-6; but see Schlotfeldt, 1987, for a fascinating article about the evolution of such definitions). The "responses" part of the definition helps to differentiate between nursing science and medical science because the medical profession is concerned primarily with the diagnosis and treatment of the health problems themselves. In conjunction with current thinking about nursing, I also include "wellness" and "illness" considerations in connection with issues of health. To take a couple of obvious research examples, a study of how the bereaved cope with the death of a close relative or friend falls easily within the definition of nursing research, whereas a study of the relative effectiveness of two different approaches to the treatment of peptic ulcers does not.

WHAT DO WE MEAN BY "QUANTITATIVE"?

As I pointed out in the preface, the modifier "quantitative" is used to classify research efforts that use traditional methods exemplified by experiments, surveys, or correlational studies of various types. Those three approaches and a few other less commonly encountered quantitative strategies are the focus of this book.

THEREFORE, WHAT IS QUANTITATIVE NURSING RESEARCH?

Quantitative nursing research is research that uses quantitative methods to advance the science of nursing by studying phenomena that are relevant to the goals of the discipline. Nursing phenomena are those facts, observations, and experiences that are the substance of nursing practice and are matters of concern when it comes to issues of health promotion and maintenance, health restoration, and health care systems.

PURPOSES OF NURSING RESEARCH

It has been argued that only research addressing clinical issues in the nursing care of individuals and groups truly qualifies as nursing research. Continuing well into the 1970s, the number of studies concerned with the profession itself, including teaching approaches and student learning experiences in schools of nursing, prompted the response that if nurses did not stop studying nurses, then the work of building a knowledge base for the discipline never would get done (see Christman & Johnson, 1981).

Currently, there are many more published accounts of clinical nursing research, that is, research conducted for the purpose of examining patients' needs, the effects of nursing interventions, or the coordination of nursing care services to patients. Although it also may be argued that research in the areas of nursing education and professionalism is inherently, albeit indirectly, concerned with patient care, the discipline is most dependent on clinical nursing research to establish the credibility of knowledge used to address nursing practice issues. In this book, I emphasize research conducted for that purpose.

Some nursing research is theory *generating,* some is theory *testing,* and some is theory *free* (i.e., it is neither directly nor indirectly connected to any sort of theoretical persuasion). **Theories** consist of sets of statements that tentatively describe, explain, or predict interrelationships between concepts. Because such descriptions, explanations, or predictions are highly valued, theory-generating research and theory-testing research usually take precedence over theory-free research.

Research that is designed primarily to extend the knowledge base in a discipline by contributing to theory generation or theory testing is called **basic research.** There are many problems in nursing and the larger field of health care that are theoretical ones. For instance, we want to extend knowledge and to better explain and understand human needs and experiences in areas such as stress and coping, social support, self-care, and ethical decision making. If we can generate research findings that lead to theory development or can design research to test theoretical propositions related to these sorts of topics, then we may be in a better position to predict and anticipate the nursing needs of individuals and groups and to plan appropriate interventions. Researchers involved in theory-based research projects need to identify their contributions to existing knowledge, as reported in the literature, in order to establish their roles in knowledge development. For example, their research might corroborate or challenge previous findings, provide new information about some phenomenon, add to accumulated evidence in some area, generate new insights, or fill an existing knowledge gap. This suggests that the research should be done with reference to a "community of scholars"—others' work (or lack of work in some cases) that, in part, determines the significance of individuals' research endeavors.

Jean Johnson's work is a good example of basic clinical nursing research. Its purpose is to extend theoretical knowledge about coping with stressful experiences associated with physical illness. There are a number of articles and book chapters that have been generated from her series of investigations of the relationship between information provided to patients undergoing various types of stressful experiences and the procedures themselves, such as surgery or radiation therapy. I suggest that you read Johnson (1966, 1973) and Johnson and Lauver (1989) for an overview of clinical studies that illustrate the importance of using theoretical explanations of coping processes when planning interventions to prepare patients for potentially stressful procedures. Then see Fieler, Wlasowicz, Mitchell, Jones, and Johnson (1996) and Johnson (1996) for more recent works.

Not all researchers investigate issues in nursing and health care from a theoretical perspective. Some become engaged in explicitly practical problem-solving research. Research that concentrates on delimited concrete problems is called **applied research**. Applied research projects sometimes may be directly connected to long-term theoretical research; in other instances, however, they may be theory free. The purpose of applied research is to arrive at pragmatic solutions to problems in clinical practice such as treatment of urinary incontinence or prevention of falls, to monitor the quality of practice in particular clinical settings, and to evaluate procedures, products, or programs. Outcomes may extend general knowledge or have a more localized impact, depending on the scope and nature of the investigation.

Some published examples of applied clinical nursing research include projects such as evaluating the validity of several blood pressure methods with stabilized adult trauma patients (Norman, Gadaleta, & Griffin, 1991), studying the effects of waterbed flotation on indicators of energy expenditure (activity level, heart rate, and behavioral state) in preterm infants (Deiriggi, 1990), and developing and evaluating a method for testing pelvic muscle strength in older women with urinary incontinence (Brink, Sampselle, & Wells, 1989).

In a practice discipline such as nursing, the difference between basic research and applied research often is in emphasis rather than in substance. That is, knowledge from basic research has both practical and theoretical implications. It can be applied to, or further tested in, practice situations. In addition, applied research findings may generate or be a part of basic research projects. The notions of basic and applied research cannot be totally disentangled. However, you may find that researchers whose projects are very theoretical as opposed to very applied have different orientations toward their works and set different priorities, even though the general repertoire of research techniques on which they draw may be the same. The purposes of the studies will determine their frames of reference. Both basic and applied approaches are essential to the discipline.

There are particular forms of investigation that are not research but use research methods, apply findings from research, and have their own special sets of methodological techniques and strategies. In the case of studies that involve quality assurance or need analysis, knowledge of research methods provides investigators with powerful tools that they can use to address practical everyday concerns arising in human service organizations and agencies. The same is true for program evaluation. Some types of evaluations are intended to advance general knowledge (and thus could be classified as "evaluation research"), whereas others are frankly acknowledged to be carried out for very specific local purposes.

DATA-GATHERING TECHNIQUES

Research methods, in their most restricted sense, are the particular techniques available to the researcher for collecting evidence (called **data** [plural] or **datum** [singular]) on phenomena of interest. For example, evidence regarding phenomena related to human behavior may be obtained in several ways:

1. Through direct observation of actions and interactions
2. Through conversation (questioning and listening to what people have to say)
3. Through examination of physical evidence (products of human behavior such as records, reports, letters, art, music, and other personal, cultural, or historical artifacts)

Techniques used in data collection include interpersonal skills involving interaction and communication styles, use of audio-visual media (audio-tape, film/videotape, photography, etc.), and application of computer technology to create and manage database systems. In the case of the natural sciences (e.g., biological phenomena), observation may need to be facilitated by the use of specialized instruments such as a microscope. Other types of data-gathering instruments include questionnaires, observation guides, and tests to measure various properties, characteristics, or responses.

WHAT IS SCIENCE?

The term "science" has been used a couple of times already in this chapter. Hardly anyone ever bothers to define it. But science is best thought of as an activity that combines research (advancement of knowledge) and theory (understanding of knowledge). A discipline may be considered "a science" or "scientific" if it has a body of theory and a body of research that is related to the theory.

Although Science = Research + Theory, not all scientists are both researchers and theorists. It is fairly common practice in many sciences for a relatively small number of scientists to do most or all of the theorizing and for the others to carry out research that either generates or tests such theories.

Some textbook authors claim that there is a process called "*the* scientific method." This method is said to include a sequence of steps that create a cycle such as the following:

1. Explore
2. Hypothesize
3. Test
4. Re-explore
5. Re-hypothesize
6. Re-test

. . . (The cycle continues and is never-ending.)

I believe that there are a number of methods that contribute importantly to the development of scientific knowledge. But I think that promotion of one approach as *the* scientific method is a misrepresentation of what it is that scientists do. The real world of science is much less structured and much more flexible than the preceding cycle suggests. It would be nice if the advancement of knowledge were that straightforward; unfortunately, it is not.

What constitutes scientific research involves different beliefs and values about knowledge and knowing, as the linguistic origins of the word "science" imply. The active discussions that continue around these ideas involve recognition of the existence of a number of different research approaches. Debates focus on the various potentials of different approaches to be combined or used sequentially in the development of new knowledge. One of the current debates concerns "quantitative" versus "qualitative" research. My personal view is that both quantitative and qualitative approaches are necessary, either together (if the goals of the research so dictate) or separately (if only one of the approaches is called for and the other would be both antithetical and counterproductive).

REFERENCES

American Nurses Association. (1980). *Nursing: A social policy statement*. Kansas City, MO: Author.

American Nurses Association. (1995). *Nursing's social policy statement*. Washington, DC: Author.

Brink, C. A., Sampselle, C. M., & Wells, T. J. (1989). A digital test for pelvic muscle strength in older women with urinary incontinence. *Nursing Research, 38,* 196-199.

Christman, N. J., & Johnson, J. E. (1981). The importance of research in nursing. In Y. M. Williamson (Ed.), *Research methodology and its application in nursing* (pp. 3-24). New York: John Wiley.

Deiriggi, P. M. (1990). Effects of waterbed flotation on indicators of energy expenditure in preterm infants. *Nursing Research, 39,* 140-146.

Fieler, V. K., Wlasowicz, G. S., Mitchell, M. L., Jones, L. S., & Johnson, J. E. (1996). Information preferences of patients undergoing radiation therapy. *Oncology Nursing Forum, 23,* 1603-1608.

Johnson, J. E. (1966). The influence of a purposeful nurse-patient interaction on the patients' postoperative course. In *Exploring progress in medical-surgical nursing practice* (pp. 16-22). New York: American Nurses Association.

Johnson, J. E. (1973). Effects of accurate expectations about sensations on the sensory and distress components of pain. *Journal of Personality and Social Psychology, 27,* 261-275.

Johnson, J. E. (1996). Coping with radiation therapy: Optimism and the effect of preparatory interventions. *Research in Nursing & Health, 19,* 3-12.

Johnson, J. E., & Lauver, D. R. (1989). Alternative explanations of coping with stressful experiences associated with physical illness. *Advances in Nursing Science, 11*(2), 39-52.

Norman, E., Gadaleta, D., & Griffin, C. C. (1991). An evaluation of three blood pressure methods in a stabilized acute trauma population. *Nursing Research, 40,* 86-89.

Schlotfeldt, R. M. (1987). Defining nursing: A historic controversy. *Nursing Research, 36,* 64-67.

STUDY SUGGESTION

Choose *one* of the articles in *one* of the present year's issues of *one* of the following research-oriented journals:

Advances in Nursing Science
Applied Nursing Research
Nursing Research
Research in Nursing & Health
Western Journal of Nursing Research

Did that article satisfy the definition of research as given in this chapter? Why or why not? If so, was it basic research or applied research? Was it a quantitative study? Why or why not?

CHAPTER 2

Research Questions and Hypotheses

CHAPTER OUTLINE

What Is a Research Question?
Some Examples of Properly Stated Research Questions
Some Examples of Questions That Are Not Research Questions
What Is a Hypothesis?
Some Examples of Properly Stated Hypotheses
Relevance for Research Design
Should Nursing Research Address Research Questions or Hypotheses?
Study Suggestions

Key Terms: research question, hypothesis

Most nursing studies are guided by research questions. Some studies test or generate hypotheses. A few have both research questions *and* hypotheses. In this chapter, I discuss the difference between a research question and a hypothesis, the phrasing of questions and hypotheses (including some good and some bad examples), and the connections between research questions/hypotheses and research designs.

WHAT IS A RESEARCH QUESTION?

A **research question** is an interrogative sentence that poses a researchable problem regarding the advancement of knowledge. All three aspects of that definition are important. First, it must actually be a question and not a statement, even though the terms "problem statement" and "research question" sometimes are used interchangeably. Second, it must be *capable* of empirical solution, whether or not the proposed study *provides* such a solution. Third, it must be unabashedly directed toward the advancement of general scientific knowledge.

Consider the following two extreme examples:

1. Nurses are good.
2. What is the relationship between age and pulse rate?

The first example is not an interrogative sentence, is not researchable, and is more a statement of faith than a matter of concern to nursing science. The second example *is* an interrogative sentence, *is* subject to empirical investigation, and *is* addressed to the pursuit of general knowledge.

It is important to realize, however, that a research question is in no sense superior to a moral claim. It may be more important for nurses to be good than for nurses to know the relationship between age and pulse rate. The issue here is merely that the former is unknowable, whereas the latter is knowable.

Although many nursing research questions deal with relationships between variables, some do not. "What is the average network size of the institutionalized elderly?" is a perfectly fine research question even though it involves a single variable (network size) rather than two variables such as age and pulse rate.

Some research questions involve theoretical concepts such as self-esteem and adaptation. Others deal with more concrete notions such as occupation and number of packs of cigarettes smoked per day. Because the purpose of research is to advance general knowledge, phrasing of research questions in theoretical terms usually is to be preferred.

Empirical evidence bearing on research questions often is evaluated for statistical significance (see Chapter 11). Nevertheless, inclusion of the concept of statistical significance in a research question is not appropriate.

Finally, research questions usually should be stated in the present tense. "What was the relationship between age and pulse rate?" sounds as though you once cared but no longer do. "What will be the relationship between age and pulse rate?" sounds as though you do not care now but may in the future.

SOME EXAMPLES OF
PROPERLY STATED RESEARCH QUESTIONS

The following research questions have been excerpted from articles that appeared in the 1995 volume of *Nursing Research*. They are illustrative of the way in which research questions should be phrased.

1. "Is there interdependence between father-infant attachment and paternal role competence among experienced and inexperienced fathers?" (Ferketich & Mercer, 1995a, p. 33).
2. "Is the influence of optimism on delay or anxiety mediated either through expectations of seeking care with a breast symptom or through perceived likelihood of breast cancer?" (Lauver & Tak, 1995, p. 203).
3. "What is the magnitude of the effect of postpartum depression on the following three subcategories of maternal-infant interaction during the first year after delivery: maternal interactive behavior, infant interactive behavior, and dyadic interactive behavior?" (Beck, 1995, p. 298).

Sometimes the research question is implicit rather than explicit. For example, Roseman and Booker (1995) stated, "The purpose of this study was to examine work factors that affect hospital nurse medication errors, including monthly changes in daylight/darkness, in an extreme northern latitude work environment" (p. 227). They could have said that the following was the research question addressed in their study: "What work factors affect hospital nurse medication errors?"

SOME EXAMPLES OF
QUESTIONS THAT ARE NOT RESEARCH QUESTIONS

1. "What is the difference between a nurse practitioner and a physician's assistant?"

2. "When was Florence Nightingale born?"
3. "Are conceptual models testable?"

These examples, which admittedly are hypothetical, illustrate the difference between a question and a research question. The first question is a matter of definition. ("What percentage of undergraduate nursing students know the difference between a nurse practitioner and a physician's assistant?," on the other hand, *is* an appropriate research question.) The second question is a matter of fact. The third question is interesting and controversial but is not researchable.

WHAT IS A HYPOTHESIS?

A **hypothesis** differs from a research question in a number of ways:

1. It is a declarative, rather than an interrogative, sentence.
2. It usually is "directional"; that is, it typically constitutes a claim (actually a guess) rather than being a noncommittal query.
3. It often emerges from some sort of theory.

Consider, for example, the research question "What is the relationship between age and pulse rate?" as opposed to the following hypotheses:

1. There is a positive relationship between age and pulse rate.
2. As age increases, pulse rate decreases.
3. Aging causes pulse rate to decrease.

All three of these hypotheses are declarative sentences, all three constitute claims about the relationship between two variables, and all three are likely to be products of careful theorizing about the aging process. The second hypothesis differs substantively from the first in that it postulates a relationship in the diametrically opposite direction (and differs grammatically in its structure). The third hypothesis is similar to the second in specifying an inverse relationship between age and pulse rate but is a much stronger—rightly or wrongly—claim because it alleges that the relationship is causal (see Chapter 3).

There are some noncommittal hypotheses (in the statistical literature, they are called "null hypotheses"), for example, "There is no relationship between age and pulse rate." But most research hypotheses are alternative hypotheses (to the null) that come from theory. Hardly anyone theorizes about the *absence* of a relationship.

SOME EXAMPLES OF PROPERLY STATED HYPOTHESES

Once again, I turn to *Nursing Research* for examples of hypotheses that are worded correctly. Here are a few, also taken from the 1995 volume:

1. "[It was hypothesized that] preschool children's social competence and behavior problems would be predicted by higher maternal depression scores obtained concurrently and one year earlier" (Gross, Conrad, Fogg, Willis, & Garvey, 1995, p. 97).
2. "[It was hypothesized that] access to Computerlink would increase decision-making confidence and skill and reduce social isolation" (Brennan, Moore, & Smyth, 1995, p. 166).
3. "[It also was hypothesized that] distress levels of husbands would be positively related to the distress levels of their wives" (Northouse, Jeffs, Cracchiolo-Caraway, Lampman, & Dorris, 1995, p. 197).

Note that although these hypotheses are stated in the conditional tense ("would be," "would increase") rather than the present tense ("are," "do increase"), they are fine. It is the tentative nature of hypotheses that often argues for use of the conditional tense.

RELEVANCE FOR RESEARCH DESIGN

If the research question, hypothesis, or purpose is properly phrased, then the choice of an appropriate research design is almost automatic. Although the specific features of various types of designs have yet to be discussed, the following chart illustrates the natural "tie-in" between certain types of designs and certain research purposes. The examples are taken from articles that appeared in the 1996 volume of *Nursing Research*.

Research Purpose	Design
"The purpose of the present study was to explore the effect of a relaxation technique on coronary risk factors while controlling for the confounding effects of dietary change, weight loss, provider contact, and the placebo effect" (Carson, 1996, p. 272).	Experiment (see Chapter 5).
"The purposes of this study were to describe the health-promoting lifestyle behaviors of employed Mexican American women and compare results with those of other published reports" (Duffy, Rossow, & Hernandez, 1996, p. 18).	Survey (see Chapter 6). As the full title of the study suggests (see reference), there also was a correlational aspect.
"The purpose of this preliminary work was to explore the relationship between nutritive sucking patterns, as a developmental assessment technique in preterm infants, and psychomotor development at 6 months of age" (Medoff-Cooper & Gennaro, 1996, p. 291).	Correlational (see Chapters 7 and 8). The word "preliminary" also suggests a pilot effort (see Chapter 15).

SHOULD NURSING RESEARCH ADDRESS RESEARCH QUESTIONS OR HYPOTHESES?

It is primarily a matter of style whether a given study uses research questions or hypotheses (or both), although there are a few things to keep in mind when making the choice. First, if there is not enough known about a phenomenon, then a hypothesis may not be able to be formulated; if there is no hypothesis to test, then a research question is sufficient. Second, in certain types of research, the hypotheses emerge at the end of the study rather than being the central focus right from the start. That is, the study is hypothesis generating, not hypothesis testing; again, questions are sufficient. But third (and finally), if the research is in an area in which a great deal already is known and theory abounds, then hypotheses are a must.

REFERENCES

Beck, C. T. (1995). The effects of postpartum depression on maternal-infant interaction: A meta-analysis. *Nursing Research, 44,* 298-304.

Brennan, P. F., Moore, S. M., & Smyth, K. A. (1995). The effects of a special computer network on caregivers of persons with Alzheimer's disease. *Nursing Research, 44,* 166-172.

Carson, M. A. (1996). The impact of a relaxation technique on the lipid profile. *Nursing Research, 45,* 271-276.

Duffy, M. E., Rossow, R., & Hernandez, M. (1996). Correlates of health-promotion activities in employed Mexican American women. *Nursing Research, 45,* 18-24.

Ferketich, S. L., & Mercer, R. T. (1995a). Paternal-infant attachment of experienced and inexperienced fathers during infancy. *Nursing Research, 44,* 31-37.

Gross, D., Conrad, B., Fogg, L., Willis, L., & Garvey, C. (1995). A longitudinal study of maternal depression and preschool children's mental health. *Nursing Research, 44,* 96-101.

Lauver, D., & Tak, Y. (1995). Optimism and coping with a breast cancer symptom. *Nursing Research, 44,* 202-207.

Medoff-Cooper, B., & Gennaro, S. (1996). The correlation of sucking behaviors and Bayley Scales of Infant Development at six months of age in VLBW infants. *Nursing Research, 45,* 291-296.

Northouse, L. L., Jeffs, M., Cracchiolo-Caraway, A., Lampman, L., & Dorris, G. (1995). Emotional distress reported by women and husbands prior to a breast biopsy. *Nursing Research, 44,* 196-201.

Roseman, C., & Booker, J. M. (1995). Workload and environmental factors in hospital medication errors. *Nursing Research, 44,* 226-230.

STUDY SUGGESTIONS

1. Did the article you chose for the study suggestion at the end of Chapter 1 have one or more research questions? Was it (were they) properly worded? Why or why not?

2. Did the article have one or more hypotheses, either in addition to or instead of research questions? Was *it* (were *they*) properly worded? Why or why not?

3. Did the type of design seem to "flow" naturally from the questions and/or hypotheses? Why or why not?

CHAPTER 3

Causality, Generalizability, and Randomization

CHAPTER OUTLINE

Causality
Other Approaches to Causality
Different Roles for Variables in the Determination of Causality
Generalizability
Randomization
Chance
How Randomization Is Accomplished
Random Assignment Versus Random Sampling
Attitudes Toward Randomization
Process Versus Product
Some Final Thoughts Regarding Generalizability
Study Suggestions

Key Terms: spurious relationship, independent variable, dependent variable, antecedent variable, intervening variable, moderator variable, extraneous variable, random assignment, random sampling, internal validity, external validity

---

Two of the loftiest goals of quantitative nursing research are the attribution of *causality* and the proclamation of *generalizability*. The most defensible way of accomplishing both goals is through *randomization*. These three topics are introduced in this chapter and are treated in more specific detail throughout the rest of the book.

CAUSALITY

Scientists always have been interested in cause-and-effect relationships. Does cigarette smoking cause lung cancer? Does stress cause depression? Does sex education cause a reduction in teenage pregnancies? But trying to determine whether X causes Y is not a simple matter.

Most authors agree that there are three conditions that are necessary for establishing that X is a cause of Y (see, e.g., Williamson, Karp, Dalphin, & Gray, 1982):

1. X must precede Y temporally.
2. There must be a strong relationship between X and Y.
3. If $U, V, W, \ldots$ are controlled, then the relationship still holds.

Consider the cigarette smoking and lung cancer example. Cigarette smoking is known to occur, or at least is believed to occur, temporally prior to lung cancer. (It is conceivable, but unlikely, that a person could have developed lung cancer before taking that first cigarette.) Therefore, the first condition usually is assumed to be satisfied. There are hundreds of studies that have shown that there is a very strong statistical correlation between, for instance, number of cigarettes smoked and presence or absence of lung cancer, and so the second condition also is satisfied. It is the third condition, however, that provides the principal stumbling block. Except for several highly controlled animal experiments in which cigarette smoking has been simulated, other factors such as genetic disposition, air pollution, and additional competing explanations have not been sufficiently taken into account for the third and last condition to be satisfied given the understandable absence of randomized clinical trials (see Chapter 5) with human subjects.

But even if all possible $(U, V, W, \ldots)$ could be controlled, all that could be justifiably concluded is that cigarette smoking is *a* cause of lung cancer, not *the* cause. Most things in this world have multiple causes, and trying to determine *the* cause of anything is a much more difficult, and usually hopeless, task.

If the first two criteria for causality are satisfied but the relationship vanishes when other considerations are taken into account regarding the third criterion, then the original **relationship** is said to be **spurious**. For example, the relationship between height and reading ability for young children is strong—the taller the child, the greater the reading ability—but it is a spurious relationship because when age is controlled, the relationship no longer persists.

OTHER APPROACHES TO CAUSALITY

It should be pointed out that although the approach to causality just described is the most common one, it is not the only one. There are at least two other ways of determining whether or not X causes Y. The first is the heavily mathematical and intellectual approach taken by statisticians and philosophers. That is beyond the scope of this book, but those of you who may be interested are referred to the article by Holland (1986) in the *Journal of the American Statistical Association* and the several reactions to that article in the same journal.

A second approach is exemplified by the determination of the reason(s) for human mortalities, which by law must be recorded on death certificates. The process is a complicated one (see World Health Organization, 1977) that usually involves an attempt to determine the medical explanation for the source of a train of events that led to a given death (the "underlying cause"). Such a determination often is accompanied by equal attention to secondary and tertiary causes in some sequential order.

DIFFERENT ROLES FOR VARIABLES
IN THE DETERMINATION OF CAUSALITY

It often is appropriate to specify different types of variables (see Chapter 10 for a precise definition of this term) that may be involved in the determination of whether X causes Y. Consider the claim that stress (X) causes depression (Y). In the traditional jargon of scientific research, stress is the **independent variable** (possible cause or predictor) and depression is the **dependent variable** (possible effect or outcome). Now consider a third variable, social support (W). It could play any of the following roles:

1. **Antecedent** (temporally prior) **variable**: Social support (or, more likely, absence of social support) might precede depression and, therefore, might also affect stress. The effect of stress on depression could actually be part of an indirect effect of social support on depression ($W \to X \to Y$).

2. **Intervening** (mediating, buffering) **variable**: Stress might lead to (a quest for) social support, which might in turn lead to (decreased) depression. The effect of stress on depression would then be indirect, through social support ($X \to W \to Y$).

3. **Moderator variable**: The effect of stress on depression might be different depending on the level of social support.

4. **Extraneous variable**: There might be some other kind of association between social support and depression; therefore, social support should be controlled when attempting to determine whether stress causes depression. (The term "extraneous variable" also includes those variables that have not been intellectualized but also may be equally defensible causes.)

There is a great deal of confusion in the literature regarding the difference between mediating variables and moderator variables. The articles by Baron and Kenny (1986) and by Lindley and Walker (1993) explained the proper distinction very nicely. (For interesting examples, see DeMaio-Esteves, 1990; Yarcheski, Scoloveno, & Mahon, 1994).

The determination of the effect of stress on depression and the role that social support plays in such a determination are used again in the chapters that follow in order to illustrate a number of issues in research design.

GENERALIZABILITY

Scientists always have been equally interested in the extent to which their findings are generalizable from the part to the whole, that is, from the sample actually studied to the population of more global interest. Does cigarette smoking cause lung cancer for everybody or just for men? Does stress cause depression only in the absence of social support? Does sex education reduce teenage pregnancies everywhere or just in New England? Finding a causal relationship that also is generalizable is the dream of many researchers. But it turns out that generalizability often is more difficult to defend than is causality.

Consider the sex education example. It is possible to study at least one aspect of sex education (knowledge of the reproductive process) in a particular setting in such a way that half of a group of pre-teens could be randomly assigned to receive such instruction and half not, with both subgroups later followed up to determine the corresponding percentages of teenage pregnancies. Suppose there were twice as many pregnancies in the subgroup that had not received instruction on the reproductive process. You would be justified in concluding that sex education was a cause (but, of course, not the only cause) of reduced teenage pregnancies *for those teens in that particular setting.* It may or may not be a cause for other people in other settings.

RANDOMIZATION

One of the most fascinating features of scientific research is the matter of randomization. It appears in a variety of forms, the most common of which are *random assignment* and *random sampling.* The purpose of the next five sections is to explore the general concept, to point out why it is so important in certain types of research, and to describe the range of attitudes various researchers have toward the principle of randomization.

Random assignment is pursued further in Chapter 5, and random sampling is discussed thoroughly in Chapter 9. The book by Edgington (1995) is particularly good for explaining the difference between random assignment and random sampling, for clarifying the role of randomization in experiments, and for understanding what sorts of statistics should be used with what sorts of randomizations.

CHANCE

Randomization is associated with the notion of chance, which in turn is based on the mathematical theory of probability. It is not my intention to delve into the intricacies of probability in this book. Most people know the probability that a fair coin will land heads is 1/2 (it is just as likely to happen as not), the probability that a man will have a baby is 0 (impossible), and the probability that all of us eventually will die is 1 (certain). So much for basic probability.

Chance has to do with the likelihood of things happening for no scientifically defensible reason other than the "laws" of probability. Results of research studies should be such that the probability of their occurrence is greater than pure chance would suggest.

The way in which the "randomization game" is played is like this. The researcher lets chance operate (e.g., by assigning subjects at random to experimental and control groups) and then determines whether or not the study findings are over and above what could be expected by chance. For an experiment concerned with the effect of cigarette smoking on lung cancer (say, for mice in simulated smoking and nonsmoking chambers), if 26% of the "smokers" get cancer and 24% of the "nonsmokers" get cancer, then the researcher undoubtedly would conclude that the smoking had no effect because such a small difference could easily have occurred by chance ("accidents" regarding which mice got assigned to which treatment) unless the sample size was very large.

HOW RANDOMIZATION IS ACCOMPLISHED

The process of randomization can be explained by comparison with a lottery. A collection of names (or numbers or whatever) is entered into a lottery, and some "unbiased" device is used to identify the "chosen" (usually few in number) and the "unchosen" (usually many in number). In scientific research, random assignment, random sampling, and any other type of randomization thought to be necessary all work in the same way. The chosen in an experiment are those who are assigned to the experimental treatment, the chosen in a survey are those who are drawn into the sample, and so on.

An important consideration is the fairness of the randomizing device. Large lotteries often rely on barrel-like containers that hold the pieces of paper on which the names or numbers are written. Small lotteries use the proverbial hat. The entries are stirred around, and one or more is blindly drawn out. It is the stirring and mixing capability that tries to ensure the fairness of the lottery, that is, to ensure that every entry has an equal chance of being a winner.

Some scientific applications of random assignment or random sampling also use barrels or hats (or coins, dice, playing cards, etc.), but the device that usually is employed is a table of random numbers. Such tables often are found in the backs of statistics books and have been incorporated into many computer software programs. The researcher attaches a number from 1 to N to each person (or hospital or whatever) in the group, where N is the total group size, and then draws n numbers from the table of random numbers, where n is the number of "winners." The table has been set up (usually by some computer-generated process) so that every digit, every pair of digits, and so on appear with approximately equal frequency. (For various ways of carrying out random assignment, see Conlon & Anderson, 1990.)

RANDOM ASSIGNMENT VERSUS RANDOM SAMPLING

Although the same table can be used for either randomly assigning subjects to treatments or randomly sampling a population, the *purpose* is not the same. We **randomly assign** subjects to treatments in an experiment because we want the groups to be equivalent at the beginning of the experiment so that if they differ at the end of the experiment, then it is the treatment that did it. In the jargon of Campbell and Stanley (1966), we want the study to have **internal validity**. We **randomly sample** subjects for a research investigation because we want them to be representative of the population to which we wish to generalize; that is, we want our study to have **external validity**.

Incidentally, the terms "internal validity" and "external validity" are poor choices because the root word "validity" is a measurement term, not a design term. (For more on this matter, see Chapter 10.)

ATTITUDES TOWARD RANDOMIZATION

Not all scientists look at randomization in the same way. "Conservative" quantitative researchers (like me) think it is absolutely crucial. They never would consider doing an experiment without randomly assigning the subjects to treatment conditions, and they never would consider carrying out a survey without randomly sampling the population of interest.

"Liberal" quantitative researchers, on the other hand, often "regard" intact groups of subjects as having been randomly assigned or sampled, or so it would appear from their writings. Most psychologists, for example, hardly ever draw random samples for their studies; their favorite subjects are undergraduate college students who take their courses. They argue, sometimes explicitly and sometimes implicitly, that people (or mice or whatever) are pretty much all alike so far as the sorts of things that interest them are concerned and that if they had drawn their subjects at random, then the subjects probably would not have differed much from the ones to which they had access. (That argument is intellectually unacceptable to conservatives.) The majority of such psychologists are less likely to apply that same reasoning in the allocation of subjects to experimental conditions; that is, they are more sympathetic to the need for random assignment than to the need for random sampling.

PROCESS VERSUS PRODUCT

It is essential to understand that the word "random" applies to the *process* and not to the product of assignment or sampling. Any device that operates in such a way that every object has an equal chance of being drawn as a winner is an appropriate randomizing device, regardless of the surprise value of the outcome. A researcher who uses a table of random numbers to draw a sample of 10 people from a population of 100 and gets all even numbers may express some concern; however, because all 100 numbers from 1 to 100 were equally likely to be drawn, there really is no reason for such concern.

SOME FINAL THOUGHTS
REGARDING GENERALIZABILITY

Even if a sample has been drawn at random, the sample findings do not constitute "proof" of a phenomenon. (That word should be stricken from all scientists' vocabularies with the single exception of mathematicians.) The findings are *evidence* in support of a particular hypothesis or claim, but even the best random sample cannot represent a population perfectly.

A second point is that it often is better to do several small *replications* of a study rather than try to answer some research question with one big random sample. (Several random samples would be best of all.) Smith may not have a random sample and Jones may not have a random sample either, but if they both arrive at similar conclusions with similar designs, then generalizability can be approximated by force of replication. (For more on replication studies, see Chapter 15.)

Generalizability also is not just a "subjects" problem. In addition to being able to generalize from a sample of people to a population of people, researchers would like to be able to generalize from the sample of measuring instruments actually used in a study to the population of instruments that could have been used, to generalize from the actual research setting to other settings, and so on. Once again, the all-purpose best way of providing a defense for so doing is randomization—random sampling of instruments, random sampling of settings, and random sampling of people.

Some liberal researchers like to argue that random sampling of settings is overly compulsive and that if a particular result is obtained in one hospital, then it also should happen in other hospitals. Conservative researchers do not agree. My favorite analogy is industrial quality control. If the inspection of a random sample of 100 widgets from Factory A yields two defectives, then you can infer that approximately 2% of all the widgets in Factory A are defective. You can infer absolutely nothing about the widgets in Factory B, no matter how similar to Factory A it may be, because you did not sample any of its widgets. That is the case not only for factories but also for hospitals, nursing homes, communities, and other settings.

REFERENCES

Baron, R. M., & Kenny, D. A. (1986). The moderator-mediator variable distinction in social psychological research: Conceptual, strategic, and statistical considerations. *Journal of Personality and Social Psychology, 51,* 1173-1182.

Campbell, D. T., & Stanley, J. C. (1966). *Experimental and quasi-experimental designs for research.* Chicago: Rand McNally.

Conlon, M., & Anderson, G. (1990). Three methods of random assignment: Comparison of balance achieved on potentially confounding variables. *Nursing Research, 39,* 376-379.

DeMaio-Esteves, M. (1990). Mediators of daily stress and perceived health status in adolescent girls. *Nursing Research, 39,* 360-364.

Edgington, E. S. (1995). *Randomization tests* (3rd ed.). New York: Marcel Dekker.

Holland, P. W. (1986). Statistics and causal inference. *Journal of the American Statistical Association, 81,* 945-960.

Lindley, P., & Walker, S. N. (1993). Theoretical and methodological differentiation of moderation and mediation. *Nursing Research, 42,* 276-279.

Williamson, J. D., Karp, D. A., Dalphin, J. R., & Gray, P. S. (1982). *The research craft* (2nd ed.). Boston: Little, Brown.

World Health Organization. (1977). *Manual of the international statistical classification of diseases, injuries, and causes of death.* Geneva: Author.

Yarcheski, A., Scoloveno, M. A., & Mahon, N. E. (1994). Social support and well-being in adolescents: The mediating role of hopefulness. *Nursing Research, 43,* 288-292.

STUDY SUGGESTIONS

1. Choose any article in a recent issue of *Nursing Research* or *Research in Nursing & Health* that may be of interest to you. Does the research report for the study refer to causality either directly (e.g., "The purpose of the study is to determine whether smoking causes lung cancer") or indirectly (e.g., "The purpose of the study is to assess the extent to which sex, age, height, and weight might account for the variation in resting energy expenditure")? If so, were all the criteria for causality satisfied? If not, should the author(s) have been concerned with causality? Why or why not?

2. Did the author(s) of that article make any generalizations from the subjects actually used in the study to some larger group of subjects? If so, were those generalizations justified? Why or why not?

3. Was any type of randomization mentioned in the article? If so, was it random sampling, random assignment, both, or neither? If not, did the author(s) acknowledge the lack of randomization, or were the data analyzed and the findings interpreted in the same way they would have been if there had been some sort of randomization?

4. Was there any discussion of antecedent, intervening, moderator, or extraneous variables? If so, were those terms used correctly? Why or why not?

CHAPTER 4

Ethical Considerations in Nursing Research

Key Terms: anonymity, confidentiality, informed consent, institutional review board

I begin this chapter by first considering the difference between nursing practice and nursing research.

WHAT IS THE DIFFERENCE BETWEEN PRACTICE AND RESEARCH?

Clinical nursing research often occurs in association with everyday practice. Research may test the effectiveness of particular interventions or evaluate the outcomes of care delivery systems. It is implemented by nurses who, in patients' eyes, are a category of caregiver on whom their safety and well-being depend. Moreover, patients and families tend to confide in nurses. Relationships of intimacy and trust are not uncommon. The same interpersonal skills required in conducting research are used by nurses to establish rapport, gather information, and diagnose and treat health problems in practice. Whether research is conducted in a care delivery setting or in participants' homes, the presence of nurses or nurse researchers is readily explained. Nurses care for patients and families in a variety of environments. They obtain access to people and are likely to be accepted in good faith because of the way in which they are involved in care delivery systems as caregivers, teachers, and patient advocates. The ethical principles involved in practice and research are the same. Consideration of patient rights, confidentiality, procedures to obtain consent, and measures to guard against risk and harm apply equally in practice and research situations.

Nevertheless, practice and research *are* different. They differ in structure, content, and purpose. Practice is directed by care plans and ongoing dialogue between members of health care teams. Research designs are guided by conceptualization of the research problem, related literature, theory, and methods of data collection and analysis.

Conducting ethical research demands that research activities be separated from those of practice and submitted as proposals for review by a panel or board of designated individuals who are prepared and empowered to evaluate the adequacy of protection of human subjects and to approve or disapprove. Activities such as testing innovative approaches or products in practice do not always constitute research. However, nurses increasingly are encouraged to introduce elements of research into their practice. If practice activities include an element of research, then they should be formally reviewed to ensure that human subjects are adequately protected.

Researchers must justify their research in terms of risks and benefits. The goal is to minimize potential risks and maximize potential benefits. Risks and benefits may be physical or psychological. When research presents physical risks, descriptions of what they may be and the steps that will be taken to avoid harm to subjects usually are straightforward. For example, in research that involves interviewing or testing, an estimate of how long and under what conditions subjects will be performing in the activity will help to determine whether sufficient care will be taken to conserve strength and energy. In the case of potential psychological risks, it may be helpful to distinguish between potential harm and personal inconvenience. The time that subjects contribute to the research and the effort expended to answer questions, take tests, perform tasks, or travel to the research site represent inconveniences that may merit some compensation. The psychological harm that could result from participation in research should be estimated with regard to what might surpass mere inconvenience and cause problems for individuals. The general safeguards built into research, such as informed consent and assurances of confidentiality, privacy, and the right to withdraw at any time without penalty, are intended to prevent anxiety about the purpose of the research and the way in which it will be conducted, to protect participants from harm, and to ensure that participation is voluntary. It is the researcher who must accept the responsibility to see that subjects are spared distress and come to no harm.

Estimation of potential benefits for subjects who participate in research is different from hoped-for benefits of the research to nursing or society in general. McCaffery, Ferrell, and Turner (1996) provided a particularly thoughtful discussion of the ethical problems involved in giving "placebos" to "control groups" in traditional experiments (see Chapter 5). The researcher must try to imagine what participation could be like from the subject's point of view. For example, many subjects are flattered to think that the researcher is interested in them or in their views on a topic. In some research projects, opportunities for individuals to solve personal problems and find support, companionship, and diversion are a byproduct of data collection. The topic of the research may have strong personal meaning or trigger altruistic tendencies in subjects, causing them to be heavily invested in helping with the project. In other types of research, subjects may be receiving direct assistance with or treatment for a problem where the individual benefits are obvious. But it is prudent to consider why anyone would want to be a research subject. (For the money? It is fairly common for researchers to give small stipends or gifts to research subjects [see, e.g., Rudy, Estok, Kerr, & Menzel, 1994; Wineman & Durand, 1992], but how do you determine whether or not to provide a financial incentive and, if so, then how much, is it taxable, and how can subjects [e.g., AIDS patients] be guaranteed anonymity if and when they are paid by check?) It is reasonable to surmise that in a thoughtfully designed project that has undergone review and offers accepted subject assurances, the possibilities for the experience to be a positive one for them are very good. Again, the conduct of the researcher will be the most powerful influence on the goodness of the research experience as perceived by participants.

ASSURANCE OF HUMAN RIGHTS

Because the care of humans is the subject matter of nursing, the protection of human rights will be a central concern in most nursing studies. Protection of human rights cannot be obtained solely from law. Human rights arise from basic needs and depend on (a) formal recognition in terms of policies, codes, and laws as well as (b) the goodwill of other humans. For example, when policies violate human rights, the avenue of higher appeal is to a concept of universal human need that ultimately resides within individuals (singly and collectively), for it is from individuals that governments and ruling bodies receive their power (Curtin & Flaherty, 1982).

Interest in the rights of research subjects has been provoked by outrage over historical incidents of human abuse in the name of science. Codes and policies regarding ethical research practices stem from expression of collective individual concerns about violations of human rights and disregard of the ethical principles of autonomy, beneficence, and justice.

A widely publicized example of controversial research practice is the Milgram experiment. In the early 1960s, Yale psychologist Stanley Milgram conducted a series of experiments on obedience and authority. The purpose of those experiments (Milgram, 1974) was to determine the extent to which people continue to obey orders when such orders conflict with their consciences. Adult subjects were recruited to "teach" a word-pairs task to a "learner" (a professional actor who was a confederate of the experimenter). Each "teacher" was instructed by the experimenter to administer an electric shock of 15 volts whenever the learner first answered incorrectly and to increase the intensity of the shock by 15 volts for each subsequent incorrect answer. In actuality, no shocks were ever transmitted to the learner, but the teacher was led to believe that they were.

The results were both interesting and disturbing. Most subjects continued to administer shocks as strong as 450 volts to the learner even when he cried out in pain, appealed for the termination of the experiment because of a heart condition, and so on. Milgram concluded that obedience to authority generally overpowered whatever moral compunctions the teachers felt and/or expressed to the experimenter.

As you might imagine, the publication of Milgram's work occasioned considerable outrage in the scientific community, prompted the introduction of additional legislation regarding the protection of human subjects in research, and led to the redoubling of efforts to establish human subjects committees on university campuses. It is indeed ironic that this study of morality, which was actually an attempt to try to understand the actions of ordinary citizens in Nazi Germany during World War II, was itself declared immoral.

The concepts of anonymity and confidentiality are associated with research subjects' right to privacy. In either case, the object is to ensure that subjects' identities are not linked with their responses. However, the two terms should not be confused. You will find that very frequently they are.

In the case of **anonymity**, research subjects are protected by the fact that their identities are not known, *even to the researcher*. This can be accomplished, for example, by the use of an anonymous questionnaire. Anonymous questionnaires do not ask for respondents' names or other types of identifiers, and they are not coded in any way that links them with individuals. Explicit informed consent is not required in such instances. Return of the completed questionnaire implies consent to participate in the study.

In cases where the identities of subjects *are* known to the researcher and others assisting in the research, subjects hardly can be promised anonymity. To protect research subjects' privacy, the researcher must ensure **confidentiality**. The promise of confidentiality must be accompanied by information about how the data will be handled. Examples of practices to ensure confidentiality include not using subjects' names or other types of identifiers in published reports of the research, grouping data when reporting results to obscure individual identities, changing details that could identify individuals and inventing fictitious names for persons and places when individual examples are needed in reporting results, keeping data in a secure location and restricting access to all but the researcher and research assistants, destroying data on completion of the research, and using data only for educational purposes. The types of measures taken may vary slightly from project to project. For example, it is not always in the best interests of the research to destroy data, but they always must be stored and accessed under controlled circumstances.

Consideration also must be given to subjects who may choose to withdraw from the research at any point after data collection has begun. Subjects need to know whether the researcher plans to use any information contributed by them before their decisions to withdraw, and they must have the option to request that the data not be used or that the data be returned to them or destroyed.

OBTAINING INFORMED CONSENT

It is essential that everyone who serves as a subject in scientific research must provide **informed consent**, either explicitly or implicitly; that is, the subject must understand what is involved and must agree to participate (see, e.g., Alt-White, 1995; Berry, Dodd, Hinds, & Ferrell, 1996). The usual device for obtaining informed consent is a consent form.

Types of information that must be printed on consent forms are noted in formal guidelines issued by the Department of Health and Human Services (1981). Such information includes the obvious factual details (title of the study, name[s] of the researcher[s], etc.) but also must address the potential risks involved in participating in the research as well as the benefits expected to the subjects themselves and/or to humankind in general.

If the research involves anonymous questionnaires, then implicit consent (return of the completed questionnaire) is sufficient, as pointed out already.

Human subjects considerations also arise in connection with the rights and responsibilities of nurses and other professionals who assist the principal investigator in the conduct of a study as interviewers, data collectors, experimenters, and the like. The American Nurses Association (1985) statement regarding the participation of nurses in clinical investigations pointed out that informed consent and other protections apply to both research workers and research subjects (see also Brown, 1996; Pranulis, 1996, 1997). Staff nurses are particularly vulnerable to subtle (and sometimes not so subtle) pressures to participate in studies that are carried out by their supervisors, and they may be exposed to risks that are over and above those associated with their usual responsibilities.

In a recent article, Douglas, Briones, and Chronister (1994) summarized the extent to which consent *rates* were reported in articles appearing in nursing research journals. Fewer than half of the articles included information regarding such rates.

INSTITUTIONAL REVIEW BOARDS

Federal oversight of procedures for regulating the use of human subjects in scientific research has developed in evolutionary fashion since 1966. At that time, the U.S. Public Health Service (USPHS) issued a series of policies concerning the establishment and function of institution-based research subject review committees, called **institutional review boards** (IRBs). Assurances of compliance with the policies were required from institutions sponsoring USPHS-funded research.

In 1974, the Department of Health and Human Services (DHHS) issued revised policies and guidelines for IRBs. A new requirement was that review boards be interdisciplinary. It was determined that competencies of the combined membership should render the ability to judge not only scientific merit of proposed research as it affects concern for human subjects but also "community acceptance" (DHHS, 1981).

In 1981, there were major revisions of the 1974 guidelines made on the basis of the report and recommendations of the National Commission for the Protection of Human Subjects in Biomedical and Behavioral Research. The revisions did not change the basic principles already laid out in earlier guidelines, but they were more specific about many procedural details associated with IRB responsibilities. In addition, they required review of all Food and Drug Administration-regulated research regardless of where it was conducted. This necessitated the formation of noninstitutional review boards (NRBs) for researchers such as physicians conducting research in their private offices who were not formally affiliated with institutions (Levine, 1986).

There are some types of research that are exempt from IRB review on the basis of no apparent risk to subjects. These include research in educational settings that involves normal education practices; research that makes use of existing documents, records, or specimens where recording and reporting information does not link individuals' names or identifiers with the data; research involving surveys, interviews, and observations of public behavior that do not identify individuals or place them at risk (not exempt when the research subjects are children); and some specific types of evaluation research that involve review of programs and procedures

(DHHS, 1981). It is important to note that individual researchers may not rule on whether studies qualify for exemption or expedited review. The classification of proposals is part of the formal IRB review process.

THE USE OF ANIMALS IN SCIENTIFIC RESEARCH

In addition to committees for the protection of *human* subjects in scientific research, since 1985, U.S. federal law and policy has mandated the establishment of committees for the protection of *infrahuman* subjects. These committees are called institutional animal care and use committees, and their charge is "to oversee the care of laboratory animals and to review scientific protocols for attention to animal welfare" (Donnelley & Nolan, 1990, p. 3).

The mistreatment of animals in research has a history similar to that of the mistreatment of humans—overly invasive procedures, unnecessary pain, crowded conditions, and, of course, lack of informed consent. The use of animals in scientific research is extremely controversial. There are three easily identifiable "camps" of opinion on the issue: (a) those (mostly medical researchers) who argue that animal research is absolutely essential for the advancement of scientific knowledge, (b) those (mostly animal rights activists) who argue that animals never should be used as research subjects, and (c) those (mostly philosophers or "the troubled middle" [see Donnelley & Nolan, 1990]) who argue for a moderate, ever-evolving approach to animal research that takes into account the potential risks to animals and the potential benefits to humans based on sound ethical principles. Just about everyone acknowledges the intellectual superiority of human to infrahuman, but the determination of the moral superiority, if any, of human to infrahuman is a very difficult problem (Rollin, 1990; Sapontzis, 1990).

There is a small fourth camp, of which I am a "member," that takes a purely statistical objection to the use of animals in biomedical research. The animals that serve as subjects in such research rarely are randomly sampled from their respective populations, and any inferences from the sample of animals actually studied to the species as a whole are hazardous at best, to say nothing about inferences to human populations. (For more on the problem of generalization from sample to population, see Chapters 3, 9, and 11.)

But even if the relevance of research on animal subjects prior to, or instead of, research on human subjects is granted (the Nuremberg Code contained a provision that *all* biomedical research on humans be preceded by research on animals), there remains the nonethical but related problem of deciding which animals should be used for which types of research. In a recent book chapter on that topic, Leathers (1990) included a long table that lists the animal group in one column, the biomedical problem for which that animal would be an appropriate model in a second column, and the corresponding specific disease(s) in a third column. For example, the first row in that table consists of the entries "mouse," "genetic/developmental defect," and "hereditary anemia." Most nursing researchers do not get involved with animal research, but for those who do, it is interesting to see which animals they choose and why.

Consider the research reported by Gunderson, Stone, and Hamlin (1991) on endotracheal suctioning-induced heart rate alterations. For their study, they used 11 Yorkshire piglets (nonrandomly sampled). Near the beginning of their article, the authors stated, "The newborn piglet was selected due to similar cardiopulmonary hemodynamics and size to the human premature neonate" (p. 139), and they cited several sources to support that choice. Leathers (1990) did not include cardiopulmonary problems in the third column of his table opposite "pig"; instead, they are listed opposite "nonhuman primates." This would appear to be an honest disagreement between equally competent scientists regarding the relevance of such research on pigs for the advancement of knowledge regarding human cardiopulmonary illnesses.

For further information on the use of animals by nursing researchers, the choice of animal model, and so on, see Westfall (1993). For an interesting example of an animal (rat) experiment that may have implications for nursing interventions regarding the healing of human wounds, see Landis and Whitney (1997) and the next chapter of this book.

REFERENCES

Alt-White, A. C. (1995). Obtaining "informed" consent from the elderly. *Western Journal of Nursing Research, 17,* 700-705.

American Nurses Association. (1985). *Human rights guidelines for nurses in clinical and other research.* Kansas City, MO: Author.

Berry, D. L., Dodd, M. J., Hinds, P. S., & Ferrell, B. R. (1996). Informed consent: Process and clinical issues. *Oncology Nursing Forum, 23,* 507-512.

Brown, J. K. (1996). Role clarification: Rights and responsibilities of oncology nurses. In R. McCorkle, M. Grant, M. Frank-Stromborg, & S. Baird (Eds.), *Cancer nursing: A comprehensive textbook* (2nd ed., pp. 1376-1387). Philadelphia: W. B. Saunders.

Curtin, L., & Flaherty, M. J. (1982). *Nursing ethics: Theories and pragmatics*. Bowie, MD: Brady.

Department of Health and Human Services. (1981, January 26). *Final regulations amending basic HHS policy for the protection of human research subjects*. Washington, DC: Author.

Donnelley, S., & Nolan, K. (Eds.). (1990). Animals, science, and ethics. A special supplement to the *Hastings Center Report, 20*(3), 1-32.

Douglas, S., Briones, J., & Chronister, C. (1994). The incidence of reporting consent rates in nursing research articles. *Image, 26*, 35-40.

Gunderson, L. P., Stone, K. S., & Hamlin, R. L. (1991). Endotracheal suctioning-induced heart rate alterations. *Nursing Research, 40*, 139-143.

Landis, C. A., & Whitney, J. D. (1997). Effects of 72 hours sleep deprivation on wound healing in the rat. *Research in Nursing & Health, 20*, 259-267.

Leathers, C. W. (1990). Choosing the animal: Reasons, excuses, and welfare. In B. E. Rollin & M. L. Kesel (Eds.), *The experimental animal in biomedical research*, Vol. 1: *A survey of scientific and ethical issues for investigators* (pp. 67-79). Boca Raton, FL: CRC.

Levine, R. J. (1986). *Ethics and regulation of clinical research* (2nd ed.). Baltimore, MD: Urban & Schwarzenberg.

McCaffery, M., Ferrell, B. R., & Turner, M. (1996). Ethical issues in the use of placebos in cancer pain management. *Oncology Nursing Forum, 23*, 1587-1593.

Milgram, S. (1974). *Obedience to authority: An experimental view*. New York: Harper & Row.

Pranulis, M. F. (1996). Protecting rights of human subjects. *Western Journal of Nursing Research, 18*, 474-478.

Pranulis, M. F. (1997). Nurses' roles in protecting human subjects. *Western Journal of Nursing Research, 19*, 130-136.

Rollin, B. E. (1990). Ethics and research animals: Theory and practice. In B. E. Rollin & M. L. Kesel (Eds.), *The experimental animal in biomedical research*, Vol. 1: *A survey of scientific and ethical issues for investigators* (pp. 19-34). Boca Raton, FL: CRC.

Rudy, E. B., Estok, P. J., Kerr, M. E., & Menzel, L. (1994). Research incentives: Money versus gifts. *Nursing Research, 43*, 253-255.

Sapontzis, S. F. (1990). The case against invasive research with animals. In B. E. Rollin & M. L. Kesel (Eds.), *The experimental animal in biomedical research*, Vol. 1: *A survey of scientific and ethical issues for investigators* (pp. 3-17). Boca Raton, FL: CRC.

Westfall, L. E. (1993). Animals, care, and nursing research. *Western Journal of Nursing Research, 15*, 568-581.

Wineman, N. M., & Durand, E. (1992). Incentives and rewards for subjects in nursing research. *Western Journal of Nursing Research, 14*, 526-531.

STUDY SUGGESTIONS

1. Choose a published research report of a study in which people were the participants and consider the human subjects aspects of the research approach described.

   a. What specific mention was made regarding human subjects concerns?
   b. If you were a member of an IRB, what information would you want to help you assess the adequacy of the protection of human subjects for such a study?
   c. If you were to conduct similar research, what steps would you take to protect the rights and ensure the safety of human subjects?

2. Choose a published research report of a study in which animals were the research subjects and answer those same three questions with respect to animals.

QUANTITATIVE
RESEARCH DESIGNS

Chapters 5 to 8 comprise the heart of this book so far as the actual designs are concerned.

Chapter 5 concentrates on the experiment, which is the traditional scientific approach to the advancement of knowledge. Although it was tempting to include in this chapter a discussion of a wide variety of specific experimental designs that have been and/or could be used in nursing research, I have resisted that temptation. There are a lot of good sources for such designs. Instead, the emphasis is placed on crucial concepts in the design of experiments and on real-world examples that illustrate such concepts.

Chapter 6, on survey research, is devoted to an approach that, on the surface, appears to be the antithesis of experimentation but, on further examination, differs primarily in specific technical details; you could actually carry out a study that is both an experiment and a survey!

The last two chapters in this part of the book, Chapters 7 and 8, cover correlational research in most of its various sizes and shapes. For convenience, Chapter 7 deals with what might be regarded as "ordinary" or typical correlational research, namely the type of research that is based on one or more correlation coefficients, whereas Chapter 8 addresses research that is equally correlational but focuses on the differences between groups rather than on the correlations between variables.

CHAPTER 5

Experiments

CHAPTER OUTLINE

Key Terms: experiment, manipulation, true experiment, experimental group, control group, empirical research, design, pretest, posttest, randomized clinical trial, quasi-experiment, placebo, repeated-measures design, double-blind experiment, main effect, interaction effect, factorial design, confounding, crossover (counterbalanced) design

I would like to begin the discussion of different types of quantitative nursing research designs with experiments because they are common to almost all sciences and because they are the best types of studies yet devised for *testing* cause-and-effect relationships. This does not mean, however, that all experiments are capable of *demonstrating* causality, as many experimental designs have serious deficiencies. It also does not mean that all research questions are amenable to experimentation. As a matter of fact, most are not, as we shall see.

In the present chapter, and in all the other chapters in this part of the book, I chose a few examples from the nursing research literature that provide prototypes of good research design for the various types of investigations with which you should be familiar. These examples are not necessarily ideal models in every respect (every study has weaknesses), but they serve to illustrate some very important points in the planning of nursing research.

WHAT IS AN EXPERIMENT?

All **experiments** involve **manipulation**, that is, the deliberate introduction of treatments (interventions), which then constitute the "categories" or "levels" of the independent variable. An attempt is made to study the effect of the independent variable on the dependent variable. For example, the independent variables of amount, type, and timing of analgesics might be manipulated so that various effects on the dependent variable, postoperative pain, might be observed. Table 5.1 provides a summary of the essential components of an experiment.

WHAT MAKES AN EXPERIMENT A TRUE EXPERIMENT?

A **true experiment** is characterized by a high degree of control over the study variables so as to eliminate the unwanted influence of extraneous variables that could affect the results of the research. In addition to manipulation, a true experiment must incorporate *comparison groups* and *random assignment* into those groups.

The use of comparison groups allows the researcher to contrast the group that receives the experimental treatment (the **experimental group**) with the group that does not (the **control group**) with regard to the

Table 5.1   Experiments Versus Nonexperiments

Experiments	*Nonexperiments*
1. Manipulation	1. No manipulation
2. Interest in the *effect* of an independent variable on a dependent variable	2. Interest in the *relationships* between variables (usually)

True Experiments
Both of the above *plus* . . .
3. Comparison groups
4. Random assignment
5. Other controls

dependent variable that is the principal focus of the research. Although the term "control group" is commonly associated with the group that receives no treatment at all, in health science research with human subjects it often is impossible not to treat or care for the group designated as the control. If the researcher wanted to assess the effectiveness of a new analgesic or a different way in which to schedule drug administration, the effects of the new treatment or intervention on subjects in the experimental group would be compared to those of the established standard procedure on subjects in the control group. The study still is an experiment, even though both groups receive medication for relief of postoperative pain. Random assignment to treatment groups is another requirement for a true experiment. Random assignment is an allocation procedure in which each subject in a study is given an equal chance of being assigned to the various treatment groups. Groups to which subjects are randomly assigned may be judged to be equivalent in a statistical sense at the beginning of the experiment, although they may not actually be equal in every respect. As the size of the groups increases, so does the probability that they are similar if random assignment has been carried out properly. (For a general discussion of random assignment, see Chapter 3.)

There are some situations in which the chance probabilities associated with the assignment to the two groups are predetermined but not equal. If the experimental treatment is very expensive, then the researcher may want to assign fewer subjects to the experimental group than to the control group, but the assignment process still can be considered to be random.

Another element often associated with true experiments that are carried out in the laboratory is the matter of environmental control. Settings that can be tailored to the needs of the research contrast with natural settings (e.g., subjects' homes, health care facilities) in which field experiments are conducted. The possibility of the intrusion of situational variables beyond the researcher's control is greater in field experiments, but the setting can be a benefit to the study by helping to place findings in their proper context and thereby permit greater generalizability.

The characteristics of a true experiment also are provided in Table 5.1.

EXPERIMENTAL VERSUS EMPIRICAL

There appears to be some confusion between the terms "experimental research" and **empirical research**. The latter term is much broader and refers to any investigation that uses data of any kind to provide some evidence regarding a research question or hypothesis. Experimental research, on the other hand, must involve direct manipulation of the principal independent variable(s) by the investigator.

PRETEST-POSTTEST DESIGNS
VERSUS POSTTEST-ONLY DESIGNS

There are two main types of true experiments: (a) those in which subjects are randomly assigned to treatment groups, a pretest is given to the groups, the subjects receive their respective treatments, and a posttest is given at the end of the study, and (b) those in which all the previous steps are included *except* the pretest. There are a number of reasons why a pretest should be part of the design. Some of these are as follows:

1. A pretest can provide some information as to the equivalence of the groups at the beginning of the experiment.
2. If probability happened to "deal you a dirty hand" and the treatment groups were quite different at the beginning of the experiment, then you can take

those initial differences into account in the analysis of the data. If there is a great deal of attrition, then you also can determine "what sorts of people" dropped out of an experiment prior to its completion. (For an example of this point, see Miller, Wikoff, Garrett, McMahon, & Smith, 1990.)

3. You can determine the change on the dependent variable from pretest to posttest for each subject in the study.

There also are several reasons for *not* having a pretest, for example, the following:

1. The administration of a pretest often can overly sensitize people to the fact that something very unusual is about to happen to them, making generalizations to unsensitized people hazardous.

2. It is more expensive to take measurements both before and after an experiment.

3. The analysis of the data is necessarily more complicated because of the additional variable.

If you are interested in a more thorough discussion of the advantages and disadvantages of pretests, then I refer you to the appropriate sections in the monograph by Campbell and Stanley (1966). They conclude that for most experiments, the arguments *against* pretests are stronger than the arguments *for* pretests.

RANDOMIZED CLINICAL TRIALS

In medical research, true experiments often are referred to as **randomized clinical trials** (Friedman, Furberg, & DeMets, 1996). The name itself is self-explanatory; it is an experiment in which a "trial" is carried out in a clinical setting for some ingredient (usually a drug of some sort) by randomly assigning approximately half of the subjects to a treatment group (they get the ingredient) and the other half to a control group (they do not). The relative effects on some dependent variable (such as whether or not death occurs) are then observed. The subjects often are infrahuman rather than human subjects (mice are a favorite choice), especially in the early stages of research on a potentially powerful drug that might have serious side effects.

Randomized clinical trials rarely employ pretests because the usual posttest (dependent variable) in such studies is whether or not mortality or morbidity occurs, and such posttests do not have pretest counterparts (for obvious reasons).

Tyzenhouse (1981) expressed surprise that randomized clinical trials have not been used more often in *nursing* research. (For recent notable exceptions, see Dodd et al., 1996; McPhail, Pikula, Roberts, Browne, & Harper, 1990; and O'Sullivan & Jacobsen, 1992.) She even coined the phrase "nursing clinical trial" and points out that the randomized clinical trial goes by several other names, for example, "clinical trial," "controlled trial," and "cooperative field trial." In a later article, Jacobsen and Meininger (1986) provided a brief history of the use of randomized clinical trials by nurse researchers and an analysis of the extent to which the reports of randomized experiments in nursing journals satisfy the standards that were established for comparable reports in medical research by Chalmers et al. (1981).

For a review of a number of issues associated with randomized clinical trials (e.g., the carrying out of smaller studies within the main study), see Fetter et al. (1989) and Hill and Schron (1992). For a discussion of sample size selection in randomized clinical trials, see Leidy and Weissfeld (1991). For a general discussion of procedures for monitoring the conduct of randomized clinical trials, see Gilliss and Kulkin (1991).

"N = 1" TRUE EXPERIMENTS

An extreme example of a true experiment is a study involving just one subject who is exposed to two or more treatments on various occasions. For example, Mr. Smith might receive 100 milligrams of Drug 1 on 10 different occasions and 100 milligrams of Drug 2 on 10 other occasions with the determination of which drug is to be administered on which occasion decided at random and with a measure taken on the dependent variable after each treatment. (Again, pretests usually are inappropriate.) Edgington's (1995) book is especially good for the design and analysis of such experiments. Holm (1983) and McLaughlin and Marascuilo (1990) provided good discussions of single-subject research in general.

RANDOM ASSIGNMENT VERSUS
RANDOM SAMPLING IN TRUE EXPERIMENTS

In Chapter 3, I explained the difference between random *assignment* (a technique used to provide control) and random *sampling* (a technique used to provide generalizability). All true experiments employ random assignment. But it is the rare experiment that also employs random sampling. The reason is that a true experiment usually involves so much cooperation by the subjects and so much attention by the investigator that a random sample usually cannot be drawn, assembled, and maintained throughout the course of the study. The consequence of this, in Campbell and Stanley (1966) jargon, is that most true experiments in quantitative nursing research have greater "internal validity" (control) than do nonexperiments but have no advantage over nonexperiments with respect to "external validity" (generalizability). Topf (1990) offered some suggestions for making nursing research more generalizable by blending laboratory and clinical settings.

QUASI-EXPERIMENTS

True experiments are highly regarded because of the extent to which extraneous influences can be controlled. There are many instances, however, when a true experiment is not feasible and a quasi-experimental design is chosen instead.

Quasi-experiments also involve manipulation of the independent variable and may use comparison groups of some sort, but they usually do not have random assignment. For this reason, serious consideration must be given to other factors that might have affected the outcome of the study. These alternate explanations are called "threats to internal validity." Quasi-experimental designs attempt to compensate for the absence of randomization in various ways. For example, one rather popular type of quasi-experimental design is the nonequivalent control group design in which two "intact" (not randomly assembled) groups of subjects are compared on the dependent variable, one having received the experimental treatment and the other not, after making certain statistical adjustments to the data that take into account differences between the groups at the beginning of the experiment. Campbell and Stanley (1966) and Cook and Campbell (1979) provided more detailed descriptions of this design and other types of quasi-experimental designs.

In spite of their limitations, quasi-experimental designs frequently are more practical in nursing research that takes place in settings less amenable to full experimental control.

PRE-EXPERIMENTS

There is a third type of experimental design called a *pre*-experimental design. Such designs are so weak that they are not worthy of serious consideration for studying cause-and-effect relationships (see Campbell & Stanley, 1966) but can be used as pilot studies carried out *prior to* primary experiments. (See, for example, the "static group comparison" design, Campbell & Stanley's Design 3, chosen by Mayo, Horne, Summers, Pearson, & Helsabeck, 1996.)

FEATURES OF CERTAIN EXPERIMENTS

Experiments often are identified according to the presence or absence of certain features in the design. As I already have pointed out, a pretest-posttest experiment involves measurement of the dependent variable both before and after the study proper, whereas in a posttest-only experiment measures are taken on the dependent variable just once (at the end of the study).

Many experiments have more than two treatment groups. The researcher may want to compare a group that gets a treatment containing the ingredient of particular interest to a group that gets an identical treatment *except* for the principal ingredient as well as to a group that gets no treatment at all. In drug studies, for example, one group may get the pill with the ingredient, a second group may get a pill without the ingredient (such a group usually is called a **placebo** group), and a third group may get no pill. In her study of postoperative pain, Good (1995) had four groups; one got a jaw relaxation treatment, one got music, one got a combination of relaxation and music, and one served as a control. In this way, the main effect of music, the main effect of relaxation, and their interaction all could be tested (see below).

There are a few experiments in which every subject is exposed to every treatment condition, usually in some randomized order. Such designs are called **repeated-measures designs.** (For interesting examples of such designs, see Baker, Bidwell-Cerone, Gaze, & Knapp, 1984, and Ziemer, Cooper, & Pigeon, 1995.)

An experiment also can have more than one dependent variable if the intervention is hypothesized to have an effect on two or more variables simultaneously.

Some experiments incorporate a "post-posttest" as well as the traditional posttest. The purpose of this is to see whether or not there are both short-run and long-run treatment effects.

Double-blind experiments (Jacobsen & Meininger, 1990) are especially desirable because for such studies neither the experimenters nor the subjects know which participants are getting which treatments. (*Somebody,* usually the principal investigator, has to know or else the data never could be sorted out!) Double-blind experiments frequently are used in randomized clinical trials, and examples of that type of experiment are provided later in this chapter. (In a *single-blind* experiment, the experimenter knows who is getting which treatments but the subjects do not.)

MAIN EFFECTS AND INTERACTION EFFECTS

In an experiment involving two (or more) independent variables, the researcher may be interested not only in the effect of each of them on the dependent variable but also in the combined effect of the independent variables. The individual effects are called **main effects,** and the combined effects that are different from the main effects are called **interaction effects.** Experimental designs in which both main effects and interaction effects are tested are called **factorial designs.**

Because the analysis of variance is the analysis most often used in controlled experiments, the terms "main effect" and "interaction effect" are very closely associated with that statistical technique.

CONFOUNDING

A term that often is encountered in experimental research is **confounding.** Confounding occurs when the effects of two or more independent variables on the dependent variable are entangled with one another. This usually is undesirable and occasionally unavoidable. If you cannot determine whether it was Variable A or Variable B that had some effect but only some hopelessly intermingled combination of the two, then the results of the experiment are, of course, extremely difficult to interpret. But confounding is very hard to eliminate, even in well-controlled experiments, because certain treatments come as "package deals" (so to speak). If Drug 1 is a pill (e.g., Tylenol) and Drug 2 is a liquid (e.g., Vicks Formula 44), then a test of the relative effectiveness of those two treatments would not be able to separate the effect of the ingredient from the effect of the form in which the ingredient is delivered.

There are situations, however, in which confounding is deliberately built into the design of the study. In investigating the effects of several independent variables simultaneously, the investigator might intentionally confound two of them (e.g., time of day and room location) because there are just too many combinations to test separately or because there is no interest in the isolation of their separate effects.

One of the very worst things that can be done in designing a two-treatment, both-sexes study is to assign all the males to Treatment 1 and all the females to Treatment 2. If those who received Treatment 1 outperformed those who received Treatment 2, then it would be impossible to determine whether it was a treatment difference, a sex difference, or both. The appropriate way in which to design such a study would be to *randomly* assign *half* of the males to Treatment 1 and the other half to Treatment 2 and to randomly assign half of the females to Treatment 1 and the other half to Treatment 2. This would produce four groups rather than two, and so the main effect of sex, the main effect of treatment, and the Sex × Treatment interaction all could be tested.

Some authors use the term "confounding variable" to refer to a variable that interferes with the principal independent variable of interest in its effect on the dependent variable and, therefore, must be controlled even if its effect is not actually studied. Room temperature is a good example; if Treatment 1 is administered in a hot environment and Treatment 2 is administered in a cold environment, then type of treatment and temperature of room are confounded.

SOME EXAMPLES OF TRUE EXPERIMENTS

I would now like to describe in some detail a true experiment that was reported recently in the nursing research literature (Wikblad & Anderson, 1995). It was a true experiment because it had manipulation, random assignment to treatment groups (but not random sampling), and other controls. The study also incorporated the unusual but very commendable feature of cost considerations as advocated by Yates (1985) and others; that is, in addition to investigating the relative effectiveness of various wound dressings, it investigated the relative costs of those dressings.

A sample of 250 heart patients were randomly assigned by Wikblad and Anderson to receive absorbent (conventional) dressings ($n = 92$), hydrocolloid dressings ($n = 77$), or hydroactive dressings ($n = 81$). [Why the n's were not all 83 or 84 is not discussed by the authors. Perhaps the variability in the n's can be attributed to the randomization procedure employed or to missing data [see Chapter 19].) The results generally favored the absorbent dressings (better wound healing and less painful to remove, although needing more frequent changes), and those dressings also were the least expensive.

Two other good examples of true experiments appeared back to back in the March/April 1996 issue of *Nursing Research*. The first, by Schilke, Johnson, Housh, and O'Dell (1996) compared the functional status of a group of 10 arthritic patients who had been randomly assigned to an 8-week muscle strength training program with 10 other arthritic patients who had been randomly assigned to a no-treatment program. The experimental group showed significant increases in all measures, whereas the control group increased only slightly during the 8-week period.

The second study, by Douglas et al. (1996), involved the random assignment of intensive care unit patients to either a special care unit or a traditional unit. The resulting mortality experiences were found to be very similar for the two groups.

Later that same year, there appeared in *Nursing Research* an article by Allen (1996) in which she reported the results of a randomized experiment involving the comparison of 59 female heart bypass patients who received a special postsurgical intervention program with 57 controls (also female heart bypass patients) who received usual care. Among other results was the important finding that members of the special intervention group decreased their fat intake, whereas the members of control group increased theirs.

Another example of a true experiment is the interesting study by Ganong and Coleman (1992) of the effect of the marital status of clients on nurses' attitudes. A sample of 83 nursing students were randomly assigned to be given information about clients who were said to be either married (Group 1, $n = 39$) or unmarried (Group 2, $n = 44$); the information provided was otherwise identical. Clients who were said to be married were perceived more positively than were clients who were said to be unmarried. A cursory reading of this article might lead one to believe that the investigation was a causal-comparative study (see Chapter 8), not an experiment. Table 1 of the article, for example, has two columns of data, one headed "married" and the other headed "unmarried" (p. 143), suggesting that the researchers studied actual clients who were either married or unmarried, which was not the case. Remember the defining characteristic of an experiment—manipulation—and you cannot go wrong.

Hanna (1993) tested the effect of a transactional intervention on contraceptive adherence. The 26 adolescent females who were randomly assigned to the experimental condition (clinic teaching *plus* the transaction intervention) had greater adherence than did the 25 adolescents who were randomly assigned to the control condition (clinic teaching only).

Campos (1994) randomly assigned 60 infants to one of three conditions for trying to alleviate heelstick pain: rocking (20 infants), pacifiers (20 infants), and control/routine care (20 infants). Both of the experimental comforting methods were found to be beneficial.

Another example of a true experiment is the study by Johnson (1996) cited in Chapter 1. Patients receiving radiation therapy for prostate cancer were randomly assigned to coping, concrete, and control groups. It was found that concrete objective information had a positive effect on mood for low-optimism patients.

Three of the most recent examples are the studies by Melnyk, Alpert-Gillis, Hensel, Cable-Beiling, and Rubenstein (1997); by Samarel, Fawcett, and Tulman (1997); and by Landis and Whitney (1997). In what they called a pilot test (see Chapter 15), Melnyk et al. (1997) investigated the relative effectiveness of two programs for helping mothers cope with critically ill children: the Creating Opportunities for Parent Empowerment program and a traditional coping program. Samarel et al. (1997) were concerned with the effects of support groups with and without coaching (they also had a control group) on adaptation to early-stage breast cancer. Landis and Whitney (1997) studied the effect of sleep deprivation on wound healing in rats. That study was referred to briefly in the previous chapter and would qualify as quantitative nursing research only under the broadest of definitions of nursing.

SOME EXAMPLES OF RANDOMIZED CLINICAL TRIALS

As I pointed out earlier, true experiments often are called "randomized clinical trials" in the health care literature. Following are brief summaries of a few nursing experiments in which the latter designation was used.

McPhail et al. (1990) were interested in studying the effect of primary care nursing versus team nursing. They randomly assigned 10 of 21 staff nurses to primary care and the other 11 staff nurses to team care, and they found very few differences between the two groups on a variety of dependent variables.

A health care program for adolescent mothers was the focus of a randomized clinical trial carried out by O'Sullivan and Jacobsen (1992). They randomly assigned 243 mother-infant pairs to either routine care (the control group) or routine care *plus* special heath care teaching (the experimental group). The most encouraging finding was that the repeat pregnancy rate in the experimental group was only 12% (after 18 months) compared to 28% in the control group.

Dodd et al. (1996) recently reported the results of a randomized clinical trial in which subjects receiving chemotherapy in each of 23 outpatient clinics were randomly assigned to be given either a chlorhexidine mouthwash or a sterile water mouthwash. Type of mouthwash was found to have very little effect on any of the three dependent variables of interest (incidence of mucositis, days to onset of mucositis, and severity of mucositis), and the water was, of course, much more cost-effective.

A trial that has received a great deal of acclaim (and some negative criticism) in the general health care literature is the Physicians' Health Study (Hennekens & Buring, 1987; Hennekens et al., 1989, 1996). This study was

Table 5.2:   Effect of Aspirin on Myocardial Infarction

	Aspirin	Placebo	Total
Myocardial infarction	139	239	378
	(1.26)	(2.17)	
No myocardial infarction	10,898	10,795	21,693
	(98.74)	(97.83)	
Total	11,037	11,034	22,071
Relative risk = 1.26 / 2.17 = .58			

SOURCE: Adapted from Hennekens et al. (1989).
NOTE: Percentages are in parentheses.

a double-blind, placebo-controlled, randomized trial designed to test two primary-prevention hypotheses in a population of healthy male physicians: (1) whether aspirin in low doses (Bufferin, Bristol-Myers Products, 325 mg every other day) reduces mortality from cardiovascular disease, and (2) whether beta carotene (Lurotin, BASF, 50 mg on alternate days) decreases the incidence of cancer. (Hennekens et al., 1989, p. 129)

It is the first aspect of the study that received national attention because the results were found to be so impressive that the aspirin component was terminated in mid-experiment in 1988. The design and the findings for that part of the experiment are discussed here. The second part of the experiment was ended in December 1995.

Approximately half of the physicians (11,037) were randomly assigned to receive active aspirin, and the rest (11,034) were randomly assigned to receive aspirin placebo. "Calendar packs" were sent to them with directions for taking one of the white tablets (both the Bufferin and its placebo counterpart were white tablets) every other day. The same subjects were asked to take a red capsule (beta carotene or placebo) on the intervening days. The results for the myocardial infarction dependent variable were the most striking. There were 139 subjects (out of 11,037) in the aspirin group and 239 subjects (out of 11,034) in the placebo group who suffered myocardial infarctions, yielding a "relative risk" ratio of approximately .58, which turned out to be statistically significant well beyond the conventional levels. Those data are displayed in Table 5.2.

This study provides a rather dramatic illustration of the difference between random assignment (which it had for a sample of 22,071 subjects) and random sampling (which it definitely did not have). The sample, although very large, may not even be representative of physicians, much less the general populace. Of 261,248 physicians who were invited to participate in the study, only 112,528 responded to the invitation; of that number, only 59,285 agreed to participate, only 33,323 were declared eligible, and only 22,071 complied with the study regimen (8.4% of the invited group).

SOME EXAMPLES OF QUASI-EXPERIMENTS

Random assignment of individual subjects to treatment conditions often is not possible because many people do not want to let chance dictate whether they will get one intervention or another. (If you randomly assign subjects to treatment conditions *without* their explicit permission, then you have a serious ethical problem.) There often is the additional issue of "contamination" when individual subjects in one treatment condition have the opportunity to interact with subjects in another condition.

The quasi-experimental design employed by Blair (1995) obviated both of those problems by using three different sites (nursing homes) to test the relative effects of mutual goal setting, mutual goal setting combined with behavior modification, and routine nursing care on self-care behaviors. (The *sites,* not individual nursing home residents, were randomly assigned to the treatments in order to avoid experimenter bias.) The combination treatment turned out to be the most effective.

A similar design was employed by Mills (1994), who gave a low-intensity aerobic exercise program to a group of elderly subjects who resided in one apartment complex and compared their subsequent muscle strength, flexibility, and balance to those of a group of elderly subjects who resided in a comparable apartment complex.

In what they referred to as a pilot study (see Chapter 15), Miller, Hornbrook, Archbold, and Stewart (1996) were unable to randomly assign all subjects to treatment conditions and had to settle for a quasi-experimental design in their study of the effectiveness of a home-health nursing intervention in providing support for family caregivers of frail elderly patients. That study also incorporated the commendable feature of cost considerations. The authors found that the cost of the intervention was lower than that of the traditional approach but that its effectiveness was not significantly better.

MATCHING

The use of "matching" in an experiment should be avoided like the plague. That term has not been used before in this chapter, for several very good reasons. How do you know on which variables to match? What constitutes a match? What do you do with the "unmatchables"? Let us consider each of these matters in turn, in the context of a familiar example such as the effect of pre-surgery teaching on post-surgery comfort.

Suppose that we decide to give pre-surgery teaching to one group and to withhold it from a "matched" group rather than randomly assigning subjects to the experimental and control groups. (Ignore, for the moment, the ethical problem of withholding information, which is a separate issue.) Do we match on sex, for example? Perhaps, but how do we know that it is an important variable? It may be that there is no relationship between sex and post-surgery comfort, in which case it would be a waste of time to insist on that matching.

What constitutes a match is no problem (usually) so far as sex is concerned, but how about a variable such as intelligence, given that the experimental subjects probably will be required to read certain materials pertaining to pre-surgery teaching? What constitutes a match there—exactly the same IQ score? Probably not, but if not, then within 5 points? Within 10 points?

Suppose that you specify *within 10 points.* What happens if you have a subject in the experimental group with a very high IQ score, say 160, and there is no one in the control group with which to match that person? Does the genius get eliminated from the study? Do you see the types of headaches that matching can entail?

Unfortunately, there are a number of researchers who continue to use matching to try to control for extraneous variables in the mistaken belief that such control is better than that provided by random assignment. Matching is attractive to those researchers who like to be "assured" that the experimental and control groups are equal at the beginning of the experiment with respect to at least one matching variable such as age, whereas with random assignment there is no "guarantee" that the groups will be comparable with respect to age. Such researchers, either explicitly or implicitly, do not trust random assignment to balance the groups on possibly confounding variables. (Some others who *do* use random assignment provide tables that contain data comparing the experimental and control groups on several variables at the beginning of the experiment, indicating that they do not trust random assignment either!) The advantages of matching in experiments are far outweighed by their disadvantages. Campbell and Stanley (1966) devoted a large portion of their monograph to very convincing arguments against matching as a means of scientific control.

THE CRAFT OF EXPERIMENTATION

Most of the discussion of experiments up to this point has centered on the science of experimentation, that is, the basic principles that can be (and are) taught in almost any good course in experimental design. Now for the craft—"pointers," insights, and suggestions that I have picked up in my work and that I would like to share with you.

The first observation that I want to pass on to you is that there is no such thing as a "pure" control group. I talked around this in brief references to regular care and to placebos, but it must be realized that in every experiment you are making a *relative* comparison. You compare whatever it is that the experimental group does to whatever it is that the control group does. In the Hennekens et al. (1989) study, for example, the control subjects did not get the ingredient that was of principal concern, but they did get *something*. (You cannot suspend a control group in a vacuum.) So, it is the "something" that is being compared to the experimental treatment, explicitly or implicitly. Had the control subjects gotten something else, the results could have been very different. The frustrating thing is that we often do not even know *what* the controls did or what else they could have done to "use up" the time that the experimentals spent getting the experimental treatment.

There is a particular type of quasi-experimental design called a **crossover design** or **counterbalanced design** in which one group of subjects gets Treatment 1 (T1) followed by Treatment 2 (T2) and another group of subjects gets T2 followed by T1. This design is a "political" favorite because if only one of the treatments should turn out to be particularly effective, then no subject will have been "left out" by being denied the benefits of that treatment. It has been suggested that a *true* experimental variation of this design might be fruitful whenever bureaucratic cooperation (e.g., by hospital administrators or deans) is a problem. Half of the experimental subjects could be *randomly* assigned to T1 followed by T2, and the other half could be *randomly* assigned to T2 followed by T1 (they would get T2 while the first group got T1 and vice versa) so as to satisfy the political concerns, but because of the possible "carryover" effects, the investigator would analyze the data only for the first treatment for each of the two groups. Half of the data would be "lost," but it would be the contaminated half, and the gain in goodwill would at least partially compensate for that loss. (For more on crossover designs, see Beck, 1989.)

Speaking of randomization, it is generally not advisable to use a coin flip to randomly assign subjects to experimental and control groups, particularly if the total sample size is rather small. For 10 subjects, for example, there is some probability that 10 coin flips would produce 10 heads, in which case every subject would be assigned to the same group. 9/1, 8/2, and 7/3 "splits" are more likely but are almost as bothersome. If you must have exactly 5 people in each group (and you really should if there are only 10 subjects altogether), then prepare a small deck of ten 3 × 5-inch index cards with the letter "E" on 5 of the cards and the letter "C" on the other 5 cards, shuffle the deck, give identification numbers 1 to 10 to the subjects, and assign Subject 1 to whatever treatment is indicated on the first card, Subject 2 to the treatment specified on the second card, and so on. (Hanna, 1993, was just lucky that her 51 coin flips resulted in 26 subjects in one group and 25 subjects in the other group.)

Another insight (I am not the only one to have this) is the constant tension between control and generalizability. Every attempt at improving control makes an experiment more artificial and, therefore, less generalizable. Carrying out a study in the laboratory rather than in the field is great for control but terrible for generalizability (unless people, such as undergraduate sophomores, behave exactly the same in a research laboratory as they do in the real world, which I doubt is the case). Randomly assigning subjects to treatment conditions also is great for control and equally terrible for generalizability. (Do ordinary people get themselves assigned to things at random?) This combination of conditions—laboratory and random assignment—is very likely to produce a "Hawthorne effect" whereby people who know they are part of a research study behave differently from how they would behave if they did not know that. One of the most important goals of experimentation is to strike a healthy balance between control and generalizability—having enough confidence in the comparability of the treatment groups but also not overdoing it so much that the research situation is completely unnatural.

So far as control is concerned, I should point out that there are at least four ways in which to control for a possibly confounding variable:

1. Hold it constant (e.g., by using only subjects who are 31 years of age).
2. "Block" on it; that is, incorporate it as a factor in the experimental design (e.g., by employing an Age × Treatment factorial design).
3. Statistically adjust for it (e.g., by incorporating age as a "covariate" in the analysis of covariance or by using the Johnson-Neyman technique [see Dorsey & Soeken, 1996; Wu & Slakter, 1989]).
4. "Randomize it out."

Suppose that you wanted to test the relative effectiveness of Diet Plan A and Diet Plan B for weight reduction but that you wanted to control for age. Holding age constant is rather simple to do but creates problems of generalizability. You could randomly assign the subjects to treatments *within* age group; that would control for age *and* permit the investigation of the Age × Treatment interaction. You could randomly assign the subjects to the treatments irrespective of age and use the analysis of covariance or the Johnson-Neyman technique to adjust for any differences on the dependent variable that may be associated with age. Or, you could simply randomly assign the subjects to the treatments and pray that probability will be good to you and that there will be little or no difference in the ages of the two groups. It is a matter of "researcher's choice."

A final suggestion: Do not ever force a research question to fit an experiment. An experiment should be undertaken only when the researcher is seriously interested in *effects* and the independent variable(s) is (are) manipulable. Questions such as "What is the effect of pre-surgical teaching on post-surgical comfort?" probably constitute, at most, about 25% of nursing research. Questions such as "What is the relationship between sex and adherence to medication regimen?" are far more common, and variables such as sex certainly are not manipulable.

This last point is absolutely crucial. Experiments are fine, but only for very restricted research questions. Most of the interesting questions in nursing research do *not* lend themselves to experimentation, yet those who pose them are as interested in causality as are those who pose the experimental ones. The problem is that the nonexperimental researchers are destined to have a more difficult time in *attributing* causality. It is tough enough trying to design an experiment that will shed some light on the effect of Pill 1 versus Pill 2 on headache relief. Trying to study the effect of stress on depression is likely to be both stressful and depressing!

REFERENCES

Allen, J. K. (1996). Coronary risk factor modification in women after coronary artery bypass surgery. *Nursing Research, 45,* 260-265.

Baker, N. C., Bidwell-Cerone, S., Gaze, N., & Knapp, T. R. (1984). The effect of type of thermometer and length of time inserted on oral temperature measurements of afebrile subjects. *Nursing Research, 33,* 109-111.

Beck, S. L. (1989). The crossover design in clinical nursing research. *Nursing Research, 38,* 291-293.

Blair, C. E. (1995). Combining behavior management and mutual goal setting to reduce physical dependency in nursing home residents. *Nursing Research, 44,* 160-165.

Campbell, D. T., & Stanley, J. C. (1966). *Experimental and quasi-experimental designs for research.* Chicago: Rand McNally.

Campos, R. G. (1994). Rocking and pacifiers: Two comforting interventions for heelstick pain. *Research in Nursing & Health, 17,* 321-331.

Chalmers, T., Smith, H., Blackburn, B., Silverman, B., Schroeder, B., Reitman, D., & Ambroz, A. (1981). A method for assessing the quality of a randomized control trial. *Controlled Clinical Trials, 2,* 31-49.

Cook, T. D., & Campbell, D. T. (1979). *Quasi-experimentation.* Chicago: Rand McNally.

Dodd, M. J., Larson, P. J., Dibble, S. L., Miaskowski, C., Greenspan, D., MacPhail, L., Hauck, W. W., Paul, S. M., Ignoffo, R., & Shiba, G. (1996). Randomized clinical trial of chlorhexidine versus placebo for prevention of oral mucositis in patients receiving chemotherapy. *Oncology Nursing Forum, 23,* 921-927.

Dorsey, S. G., & Soeken, K. L. (1996). Use of the Johnson-Neyman technique as alternative to analysis of covariance. *Nursing Research, 45,* 363-366.

Douglas, S., Daly, B. J., Rudy, E. B., Sereika, S. M., Menzel, L., Song, R., Dyer, M. A., & Mintenegor, H. D. (1996). Survival experience of chronically critically ill patients. *Nursing Research, 45,* 73-77.

Edgington, E. S. (1995). *Randomization tests* (3rd ed.). New York: Marcel Dekker.

Fetter, M. S., Feetham, S. L., D'Apolito, K., Chaze, B. A., Fink, A., Frink, B. B., Hougart, M. K., & Rushton, C. H. (1989). Randomized clinical trials: Issues for researchers. *Nursing Research, 38,* 117-120.

Friedman, L. M., Furberg, C. D., & DeMets, D. L. (1996). *Fundamentals of clinical trials* (3rd ed.). St. Louis, MO: Mosby.

Ganong, L. H., & Coleman, M. (1992). The effect of clients' family structure on nursing students' cognitive schemas and verbal behavior. *Research in Nursing & Health, 15,* 139-146.

Gilliss, C. L., & Kulkin, I. L. (1991). Monitoring nursing interventions and data collection in a randomized clinical trial. *Western Journal of Nursing Research, 13,* 416-422.

Good, M. (1995). A comparison of the effects of jaw relaxation and music on postoperative pain. *Nursing Research, 44,* 52-57.

Hanna, K. (1993). Effect of nurse-client transaction on female adolescents' oral contraceptive adherence. *Image, 25,* 285-290.

Hennekens, C. H., & Buring, J. E. (1987). *Epidemiology in medicine.* Boston: Little, Brown.

Hennekens, C. H., Buring, J. E., Manson, J. E., Stampfer, M., Rosner, B., Cook, N. R., Belanger, C., LaMotte, F., Gaziano, J. M., Ridker, P. M., Willett, W., & Peto, R. (1996). Lack of evidence of long-term supplementation with beta carotene on the incidence of malignant neoplasms and cardiovascular disease. *New England Journal of Medicine, 334,* 1145-1149.

Hennekens, C. H., et al. for members of the Steering Committee of the Physicians' Health Study Research Group. (1989). Final report on the aspirin component of the ongoing Physicians' Health Study. *New England Journal of Medicine, 321,* 129-135.

Hill, M. N., & Schron, E. B. (1992). Opportunities for nurse researchers in clinical trials. *Nursing Research, 41,* 114-116.

Holm, K. (1983). Single subject research. *Nursing Research, 32,* 253-255.

Jacobsen, B. S., & Meininger, J. C. (1986). Randomized experiments in nursing: The quality of reporting. *Nursing Research, 35,* 379-382.

Jacobsen, B. S., & Meininger, J. C. (1990). Seeing the importance of blindness. *Nursing Research, 39,* 54-57.

Johnson, J. E. (1996). Coping with radiation therapy: Optimism and the effect of preparatory interventions. *Research in Nursing & Health, 19,* 3-12.

Landis, C. A., & Whitney, J. D. (1997). Effects of 72 hours sleep deprivation on wound healing in the rat. *Research in Nursing & Health, 20,* 259-267.

Leidy, N. K., & Weissfeld, L. A. (1991). Sample sizes and power computation for clinical intervention trials. *Western Journal of Nursing Research, 13,* 138-144.

Mayo, D. J., Horne, M. K., III, Summers, B. L., Pearson, D. C., & Helsabeck, C. B. (1996). The effects of heparin flush on patency of the Groshong catheter. *Oncology Nursing Forum, 23,* 1401-1405.

McLaughlin, F. E., & Marascuilo, L. A. (1990). *Advanced nursing and health care research: Quantification approaches.* Philadelphia: W. B. Saunders.

McPhail, A., Pikula, H., Roberts, J., Browne, G., & Harper, D. (1990). Primary nursing: A randomized crossover trial. *Western Journal of Nursing Research, 12,* 188-200.

Melnyk, B. M., Alpert-Gillis, L. J., Hensel, P. B., Cable-Beiling, R. C., & Rubenstein, J. S. (1997). Helping mothers cope with a critically ill child: A pilot test of the COPE intervention. *Research in Nursing & Health, 20,* 3-14.

Miller, L. L., Hornbrook, M. C., Archbold, P. G., & Stewart, B. J. (1996). Development of use and cost measures in a nursing intervention for family caregivers and frail elderly patients. *Research in Nursing & Health, 19,* 273-285.

Miller, P., Wikoff, R., Garrett, M. J., McMahon, M., & Smith, T. (1990). Regimen compliance two years after myocardial infarction. *Nursing Research, 39,* 333-336.

Mills, E. M. (1994). The effect of low-intensity aerobic exercise on muscle strength, flexibility, and balance among sedentary elderly persons. *Nursing Research, 43,* 207-211.

O'Sullivan, A. L., & Jacobsen, B. S. (1992). A randomized trial of a health care program for first-time adolescent mothers and their infants. *Nursing Research, 41,* 210-215.

Samarel, N., Fawcett, J., & Tulman, L. (1997). Effect of support groups with coaching on adaptation to early stage breast cancer. *Research in Nursing & Health, 20,* 15-26.

Schilke, J. M., Johnson, G. O., Housh, T. J., & O'Dell, J. R. (1996). Effects of muscle-strength training on the functional status of patients with osteoarthritis of the knee joint. *Nursing Research, 45,* 68-72.

Topf, M. (1990). Increasing the validity of research results with a blend of laboratory and clinical strategies. *Image, 22,* 121-123.

Tyzenhouse, P. S. (1981). The nursing clinical trial. *Western Journal of Nursing Research, 3*, 102-109.

Wikblad, K., & Anderson, B. (1995). A comparison of three wound dressings in patients undergoing heart surgery. *Nursing Research, 44*, 312-316.

Wu, Y.-W. B., & Slakter, M. J. (1989). Analysis of covariance in nursing research. *Nursing Research, 38*, 306-308.

Yates, M. A. (1985). Cost savings as an indicator of successful nursing intervention. *Nursing Research, 34*, 50-53.

Ziemer, M. M., Cooper, D. M., & Pigeon, J. G. (1995). Evaluation of a dressing to reduce nipple pain and improve nipple skin condition in breast-feeding women. *Nursing Research, 44*, 347-351.

STUDY SUGGESTIONS

1. Choose a recent issue of one of the general nursing research journals (e.g., *Nursing Research, Research in Nursing & Health*) or one of the specialized nursing research journals (e.g., *Heart & Lung, Oncology Nursing Forum*), read the first article in that issue, and answer the following questions:

    a. Is the research reported in the article an experiment? Why?

    b. If so, . . .

        (i) Is it a true experiment or a quasi-experiment? Why or why not?

        (ii) Is there a pretest? If so, was it really needed? If not, do you think there should have been one? Why or why not?

    c. Does the study have random sampling? Random assignment? Both? Neither? What are the implications of the presence or absence of those features?

2. Phrase a research hypothesis of interest to you. (For help in phrasing a research hypothesis, see Chapter 2.) Then answer the following questions:

    a. Would a true experiment be appropriate for providing evidence regarding that hypothesis? Why or why not?

    b. If so, what sort of design would you employ? Would you include a pretest? Why or why not? Would you be interested in both main and interaction effects? Why or why not?

Surveys

WHAT IS A SURVEY?

The American Statistical Association (varying dates) publishes a small pamphlet that carries this very title. Approximately half of the scientific community seems to define survey research as any research that involves questionnaires and/or interviews for large numbers of respondents. Others define survey research as any research based on a probability sample, that is, a sample drawn from a population in such a way that every subject has a known probability of being selected. (The term "sample survey" sometimes is used in conjunction with this second definition.)

Surveys that are based on probability samples may or may not involve questionnaires or interviews and may or may not involve large numbers of participants. For example, a study in which a simple random sample of 29 adult males have their temperatures taken would be regarded by some people as a survey, whereas others would call that sort of study something else. ("Descriptive research" is a popular catch-all term.)

Surveys usually are conducted for the general purpose of obtaining information about practices, opinions, attitudes, and other characteristics of people. Survey researchers typically collect a broad range of demographic data on participants' backgrounds as well. Although these data may not be central to the study, they may help to interpret the study findings, given that personal and environmental characteristics frequently can be linked with behavioral and attitudinal patterns. The most basic function of a survey is description, although explanation (of why people behave or believe as they do), comparison, and prediction of responses with regard to the variable(s) of interest may be additional objectives.

A number of data collection techniques may be used in surveys. (Hash, Donlea, & Walljasper, 1985, for example, argued for greater use of telephone interviews for nursing surveys rather than relying on mailed questionnaires.) But the main concerns are with sampling procedures, sample size, and instrument validity and reliability. The researcher tries to obtain as large a sample as feasible to keep sampling error at a minimum and to allow for a certain percentage of nonresponse. Careful construction of questionnaires or interview schedules and pilot testing of these instruments are important. A pilot study based on a small preliminary sample can alert the researcher to questions that may need to be changed or deleted or to additional questions that should be included. (For some additional concerns regarding the use of questionnaires, especially mailed questionnaires, see Topf, 1986a, and Woolley, 1984.)

An advantage of surveys is that large amounts of data can be amassed. A disadvantage is that the actual information content might be fairly superficial. The researcher must determine whether study interests are best served by an extensive survey focused on selected variables or by an intensive examination of more variables with a smaller sample or even a single subject. Because the survey researcher usually has little control over the research situation, causal relationships are more difficult to establish and may not even be of primary interest. However, carefully designed surveys can be objective, are a good source for hypotheses, and can suggest directions for further research.

As already suggested, surveys "rise or fall" on sampling and measurement considerations. Two later chapters in this text deal explicitly with such matters. Chapter 9 discusses basic concepts in sampling, various types of sampling designs, and sample size determination. Chapter 10 addresses a number of measurement issues. To avoid unnecessary duplication, the present chapter concentrates on examples of nursing research surveys. I have chosen five studies that are surveys in both senses of the term; that is, they were based on probability samples *and* they used questionnaires or interviews. The sixth example is a study based on a probability sample, but it did not involve questionnaires or interviews. The final two examples used questionnaires but were based on nonprobability samples.

EXAMPLES OF SURVEYS IN NURSING RESEARCH

Two examples of surveys that fit both of the competing definitions and also are substantively similar to one another are the studies by Smith and Shamansky (1983) and Shamansky, Schilling, and Holbrook (1985) of the market for nurse practitioner services in Seattle, Washington, and New Haven, Connecticut, respectively. The Seattle study was a telephone survey of a stratified random sample of 239 residents who were asked a variety of questions about their interest in taking advantage of family nurse practitioner services. The New Haven study was a telephone survey of a larger stratified random sample of residents ($N = 331$) who were asked similar questions about general nurse practitioner services.

Another example of a survey that involved both probability sampling and a questionnaire is the study by Wagner (1985) of the smoking behavior of a sample of nurses in New York State. Using a mailing list of 16,125 registered nurses who were licensed in New York and who lived in one of the seven counties in the western part of that state, Wagner sent out questionnaires to a 5% random sample of that population. Approximately 62% of those who received the questionnaires ($n = 504$) responded after two follow-up mailings. This study provides an excellent illustration of the four "layers" of any sampling plan (see Chapter 9): the target population (all nurses in the United States), the sampled population (the 16,125 nurses on the mailing list), the drawn sample (5% of that list), and the responding sample (the 504 nurses who actually mailed back their questionnaires). The author would have liked to generalize his findings (e.g., that 28% of nurses were current smokers) from the responding sample to the target population, but because the target population was not the population that was actually sampled and because the response rate was only 62%, he was not able to do so.

A related study was the survey of substance abuse by nurses carried out by Trinkoff, Eaton, and Anthony (1991), which also involved a comparison between nurses and non-nurses. (For an extended discussion of this study, see Chapter 8.)

A fifth example of survey research that also fits both definitions is the study by Pender and Pender (1986). They were interested in a number of variables such as attitudes toward exercise and diet and the avoidance of stressful situations. Their sampling plan was a complicated one, incorporating several stages (again, see Chapter 9): city blocks, houses, and individual respondents. Individual interviews were held in the homes using a 75-item structured questionnaire. A total sample of 377 persons was realized, and the statistical procedure known as stepwise multiple regression analysis (see Chapter 11) was used to test various hypotheses arising from the theory of "reasoned action."

Ballard and McNamara (1983) carried out a retrospective survey of 397 records of cardiac and cancer patients in Connecticut who had received home health care by various agencies. The purpose of their study was to determine the nursing needs of such patients. They explicitly defined their target population as "all patients with a diagnosis of cancer or cardiac disease who were discharged from a home health care agency in 1979 or 1980" (p. 237). Using a very complicated but highly commendable sampling design, they carefully studied the records of 174 men and 223 women ranging in age from 1 to 96 years, identified a health status score (a measure of deficiencies in daily activities and severity of nursing problems) as the strongest predictor of the need for agency visits, and made a number of recommendations for future research on home health care.

The most recent article (as of the end of 1997) was by Huang et al. (1997) on the relationship between weight and the risk of breast cancer. One of the other recent examples of survey research regarding the use of questionnaires is the study by Miller and Champion (1996) of self-reported mammography for a nonprobability sample of 1,083 older women (age 50 years or older). This study also had a correlational aspect (see Chapters 7 and 8) in that a number of relationships between mammography use and other variables (satisfaction with way of living, perceived benefits of mammography, etc.) also were explored.

An example of a survey that involves lots of questionnaires and a large nonprobability sample is the ongoing Nurses' Health Study, which is under the same auspices as the Physicians' Health Study (Hennekens et al., 1989, 1996; see Chapter 5). The Nurses' Health Study is arguably medical research or sociological research rather than nursing research (epidemiologists probably would call it a prospective observational study), and its findings have been published in a variety of non-nursing journals; however, because all the subjects participating in the study are nurses, it should be of considerable interest to nursing researchers. The first article was written by Hennekens et al. (1979) and dealt with the association between hair dyes and cancer (they found none) for a sample of 120,557 nurses. One of the most recent publications based on that study (Seddon, Willett, Speizer, & Hankinson, 1996) addressed the relationship between cigarette smoking and macular degeneration. Interestingly, the article immediately following that one in the *Journal of the American Medical Association* reported the results of an almost identical study of subjects who participated in the Physicians' Health Study (see Christen, Glynn, Manson, Ajani, & Buring, 1996). Both studies found a weak but statistically significant relationship.

Because the Nurses' Health Study has a number of fascinating features so far as research design is concerned, I devote the remainder of this chapter to a critical examination of some of those features and the implications of such an examination for quantitative nursing research in general.

THE NURSES' HEALTH STUDY: KUDOS AND BRICKBATS

The study has many positive aspects. First, and perhaps most obvious, is the very impressive sample size. The mere drawing of such a sample, from a 1972 inventory conducted by the American Nurses Association, must have been a tremendous undertaking in and of itself.

Second, the response (participation) rate has been phenomenal compared to those in other similar surveys. Of the 172,413 registered nurses in 11 states (more about this later) to whom questionnaires were mailed at the beginning of the study, completed forms were received from about 121,000 of them (approximately 70%). Contrast that with the response rate for the Physicians' Health Study (Hennekens et al., 1989, 1996) of only 8% (22,071 out of 261,248). Most nursing research studies have response rates somewhere between the two.

What is even more amazing and commendable is the continued participation rate. The initial questionnaires were mailed out in 1976, and subsequent questionnaires were mailed out every 2 years thereafter. Some of the follow-up rates were 89% in 1978, 85% in 1980, and 95% in 1982 (the latter figure included some additional telephoning); the most recent follow-up rate that has been reported (as of 1992) was more than 90% (Seddon et al., 1996).

A fourth aspect of this study worthy of praise was the researchers' attempt to ascertain which of the subjects died during each questionnaire cycle. By an exhaustive search of vital records and the National Death Index, they claimed (Stampfer et al., 1984) to have correctly identifed more than 98% of subject deaths as of 1984.

A fifth and final (for now, anyhow) kudo, which also has an associated brickbat, goes to the research team for its attempt to validate the responses given by the nurses to certain items on the questionnaires. Several of the research team's published articles deal with this matter (e.g., Colditz et al., 1986; Colditz, Willett, Stampfer, Rosner, et al., 1987; Colditz, Willett, Stampfer, Sampson, et al., 1987). The research team members were particularly concerned about the accuracy of the information regarding age, smoking behavior, alcohol intake, onset of menopause, and a few other variables, and so they sought and received permission from some of the subjects to gain access to their medical records to corroborate the subjects' self-reports. (The agreement was very good.)

The matter of "validation," "confirmation," "corroboration," or what these researchers sometimes call "reproducibility" (corroboration is the safest term because agreement does not necessarily imply truth) brings us to the first of several bothersome aspects of the Nurses' Health Study—the lack of anonymity and the accompanying invasion of privacy that characterize much of this investigation. In typical questionnaire research, the responding subjects can answer freely and honestly because they usually are assured of both anonymity (you will never be known by name) and confidentiality (your responses will be privileged information). Whenever a specific response can be identified with a particular respondent by name, serious ethical questions arise (see Chapter 4). On the other hand, it can be argued that nobody forced the respondents to identify themselves and to give permission to study their medical records; so, in that respect, everything appears to be open and above board. I remain concerned.

A second negative aspect of this study is the decision to concentrate on the population of registered nurses in only 11 of the 50 states (California,

Connecticut, Florida, Maryland, Massachusetts, Michigan, New Jersey, New York, Ohio, Pennsylvania, and Texas). Those nurses may not be representative of registered nurses in general. As a matter of fact, the population initially was restricted to "all married, female, registered nurses born between 1921 and 1946" (Hennekens et al., 1979, p. 1391) who were living in those states in 1972 and who may, therefore, be even less representative.

Worse yet, those 121,000 nurses usually are taken to be representative of all *women*. (The 22,071 physicians in the Physicians' Health Study also are taken to be representative of all men!) Nurses are likely to be healthier and better educated than women in general, but they also are likely to be under greater stress. Although the first report by Hennekens et al. in *The Lancet* in 1979 was titled "Use of Permanent Hair Dyes and Cancer Among *Registered Nurses*" (emphasis added), subsequent articles bore titles such as "Relative Weight and Risk of Breast Cancer Among Premenopausal *Women*" (Willett et al., 1985, emphasis added); "Validation of Questionnaire Information on Risk Factors and Disease Outcomes in a Prospective Cohort Study of *Women*" (Colditz et al., 1986, emphasis added); "A Prospective Study of Age at Menarche, Parity, Age at First Birth, and Coronary Heart Disease in *Women*" (Colditz, Stampfer, et al., 1987, emphasis added); "Cigarette Smoking and Risk of Stroke in Middle-Aged *Women*" (Colditz et al., 1988, emphasis added); "Weight, Weight Change, and Coronary Heart Disease in *Women*" (Willett et al., 1995, emphasis added); "The Use of Estrogens and Progestins and the Risk of Breast Cancer in Postmenopausal *Women*" (Colditz et al., 1995, emphasis added); "Body Weight and Mortality Among *Women*" (Manson et al., 1995, emphasis added); "Coffee Consumption and Coronary Heart Disease in *Women*" (Willett et al., 1996, emphasis added); "A Prospective Study of Cigarette Smoking and Age-Related Macular Degeneration in *Women*" (Seddon et al., 1996, emphasis added); and "Dietary Fiber, Glycemic Load, and Risk of Non-Insulin-Dependent Diabetes Mellitus in *Women*" (Salmeron et al., 1997, emphasis added). Five of the reports (Colditz et al., 1993; Huang et al., 1997; Kawachi et al., 1997; Sanchez-Guerrero et al., 1995; Stampfer et al., 1991) avoided the problem by using the titles "Family History, Age, and Risk of Breast Cancer," "Dual Effects of Weight and Weight Gain on Breast Cancer Risk," "A Prospective Study of Passive Smoking and Coronary Heart Disease," "Silicone Breast Implants and the Risk of Connective-Tissue Diseases and Symptoms," and "Postmenopausal Estrogen Therapy and Cardiovascular Disease," respectively. (For a defense of why they chose nurses and not a more representative sample of women, see Hennekens & Buring, 1987, p. 38.)

One final negative criticism of this study: Unless I am mistaken regarding the backgrounds of the members of the research team, no one is a nurse researcher. If you are going to study nurses, then it would be prudent to have at least one person on the research team who has both an R.N. and a Ph.D. Perhaps in partial atonement for this oversight, the authors of the report on obesity and coronary heart disease (Manson et al., 1990) did at least express their indebtedness to the registered nurses who were the study subjects!

IMPLICATIONS

What can be learned from this critique of the Nurses' Health Study? On the positive side, we know that it is possible to obtain the cooperation of very large numbers of subjects for survey research and to maintain their interest in continuing to participate over extended periods of time. On the negative side, we must exercise caution in generalizing from a sample of nurses to all women and in "outwearing our welcome" by subordinating considerations of anonymity and confidentiality to a concern for corroboration of self-reports and completeness of data. Did the Colditz team go too far? I am inclined to think that they did, but I urge you to read some or all of the reports of the Nurses' Health Study and decide for yourself.

A FINAL NOTE

Three surveys that should be of considerable interest to nursing researchers are the National Health and Nutrition Examination Survey, the National Health Interview Survey, and the National Survey of Families and Households. The first two are not actually survey research as such, but the information collected in those surveys can be used for research purposes. The latter survey has as its primary purpose the advancement of general knowledge regarding various living arrangements, and it is treated in greater detail in the chapter on secondary analysis (Chapter 13).

REFERENCES

American Statistical Association. (varying dates). *What is a survey?* Washington, DC: Author.

Ballard, S., & McNamara, R. (1983). Quantifying nursing needs in home health care. *Nursing Research, 32,* 236-241.

Christen, W. G., Glynn, R. J., Manson, J. E., Ajani, U. A., & Buring, J. E. (1996). A prospective study of cigarette smoking and risk of age-related macular degeneration in men. *Journal of the American Medical Association, 276,* 1147-1151.

Colditz, G. A., Bonita, R., Stampfer, M. J., Willett, W. C., Rosner, B., Speizer, F. E., & Hennekens, C. H. (1988). Cigarette smoking and risk of stroke in middle-aged women. *New England Journal of Medicine, 318,* 937-941.*

Colditz, G. A., Hankinson, S. E., Hunter, D. J., Willett, W. C., Manson, J. E., Stampfer, M. J., Hennekens, C. H., Rosner, B., & Speizer, F. E. (1995). The use of estrogens and progestins and the risk of breast cancer in postmenopausal women. *New England Journal of Medicine, 332,* 1589-1593.*

Colditz, G. A., Martin, P., Stampfer, M. J., Willett, W. C., Sampson, L., Rosner, B., Hennekens, C. H., & Speizer, F. E. (1986). Validation of questionnaire information on risk factors and disease outcomes in a prospective cohort of women. *American Journal of Epidemiology, 123,* 894-900.*

Colditz, G. A., Stampfer, M. J., Willett, W. C., Stason, W. B., Rosner, B., Hennekens, C. H., & Speizer, F. E. (1987). Reproducibility and validity of self-reported menopausal status in a prospective cohort study. *American Journal of Epidemiology, 126,* 319-325.*

Colditz, G. A., Willett, W. C., Hunter, D. J., Stampfer, M. J., Manson, J. E., Hennekens, C. H., Rosner, B. A., & Speizer, F. E. (1993). Family history, age, and risk of breast cancer. *Journal of the American Medical Association, 270,* 338-343.*

Colditz, G. A., Willett, W. C., Stampfer, M. J., Rosner, B., Speizer, F. E., & Hennekens, C. H. (1987). A prospective study of age at menarche, parity, age at first birth, and coronary heart disease in women. *American Journal of Epidemiology, 126,* 861-870.*

Colditz, G. A., Willett, W. C., Stampfer, M. J., Sampson, M. J., Rosner, B., Hennekens, C. H., & Speizer, F. E. (1987). The influence of age, relative weight, smoking, and alcohol intake on the reproducibility of a dietary questionnaire. *International Journal of Epidemiology, 16,* 392-398.*

Hash, V., Donlea, J., & Walljasper, D. (1985). The telephone survey: A procedure for assessing educational needs of nurses. *Nursing Research, 34,* 126-128.

Hennekens, C. H., & Buring, J. E. (1987). *Epidemiology in medicine.* Boston: Little, Brown.

Hennekens, C. H., Buring, J. E., Manson, J. E., Stampfer, M., Rosner, B., Cook, N. R., Belanger, C., LaMotte, F., Gaziano, J. M., Ridker, P. M., Willett, W., & Peto, R. (1996). Lack of evidence of long-term supplementation with beta carotene on the incidence of malignant neoplasms and cardiovascular disease. *New England Journal of Medicine, 334,* 1145-1149.

Hennekens, C. H., Rosner, B., Belanger, C., Speizer, F. E., Bain, C. J., & Peto, R. (1979). Use of permanent hair dyes and cancer among registered nurses. *Lancet, 79*(2), 1390-1393.

Hennekens, C. H., et al. for members of the Steering Committee of the Physicians' Health Study Research Group. (1989). Final report on the aspirin component of the ongoing Physicians' Health Study. *New England Journal of Medicine, 321,* 129-135.

Huang, Z., Hankinson, S. E., Colditz, G. A., Stampfer, M. J., Hunter, D. J., Manson, J. E., Hennekens, C. H., Rosner, B., Speizer, F. E., & Willett, W. C. (1997). Dual effects of

AUTHOR'S NOTE: * = Nurses' Health Study.

weight and weight gain on breast cancer risk. *Journal of the American Medical Association, 278,* 1407-1449.*

Kawachi, I., Colditz, G. A., Speizer, F. E., Manson, J. E., Stampfer, M. J., Willett, W. C., & Hennekens, C. H. (1997). A prospective study of passive smoking and coronary heart disease. *Circulation, 95,* 2374-2379.*

Manson, J. E., Colditz, G. A., Stampfer, M. J., Willett, W. C., Rosner, B., Monson, R. R., Speizer, F. E., & Hennekens, C. H. (1990). A prospective study of obesity and risk of coronary heart disease in women. *New England Journal of Medicine, 322,* 882-889.*

Manson, J. E., Willett, W. C., Stampfer, M. J., Colditz, G. A., Hunter, D. J., Hankinson, S. E., Hennekens, C. H., & Speizer, F. E. (1995). Body weight and mortality among women. *New England Journal of Medicine, 333,* 677-685.*

Miller, A. M., & Champion, V. L. (1996). Mammography in older women: One-time and three-year adherence to guidelines. *Nursing Research, 45,* 239-245.

Pender, N. J., & Pender, A. R. (1986). Attitudes, subjective norms, and intentions to engage in health behaviors. *Nursing Research, 35,* 15-18.

Salmeron, J., Manson, J. E., Stampfer, M. J., Colditz, G. A., Wing, A. L., & Willett, W. C. (1997). Dietary fiber, glycemic load, and risk of non-insulin-dependent diabetes mellitus in women. *Journal of the American Medical Association, 277,* 472-477.*

Sanchez-Guerrero, J., Colditz, G. A., Karlson, E. W., Hunter, D. J., Speizer, F. E., & Liang, M. H. (1995). Silicone breast implants and the risk of connective-tissue diseases and symptoms. *New England Journal of Medicine, 332,* 1666-1670.*

Seddon, J. M., Willett, W. C., Speizer, F. E., & Hankinson, S. E. (1996). A prospective study of cigarette smoking and age-related macular deterioration in women. *Journal of the American Medical Association, 276,* 1141-1146.*

Shamansky, S. L., Schilling, L. S., & Holbrook, T. L. (1985). Determining the market for nurse practitioner services: The New Haven experience. *Nursing Research, 34,* 242-247.

Smith, D. W., & Shamansky, S. L. (1983). Determining the market for family nurse practitioner services: The Seattle experience. *Nursing Research, 32,* 301-305.

Stampfer, M. J., Colditz, G. A., Willett, W. C., Manson, J. E., Rosner, B., Speizer, F. E., & Hennekens, C. H. (1991). Postmenopausal estrogen therapy and cardiovascular disease. *New England Journal of Medicine, 325,* 756-762.*

Stampfer, M. J., Willett, W. C., Speizer, F. E., Dysert, D. C., Lipnick, R., Rosner, B., & Hennekens, C. H. (1984). Test of the National Death Index. *American Journal of Epidemiology, 119,* 837-839.*

Topf, M. (1986a). Response sets in questionnaire research. *Nursing Research, 35,* 119-121.

Trinkoff, A. M., Eaton, W. W., & Anthony, J. C. (1991). The prevalence of substance abuse among registered nurses. *Nursing Research, 40,* 172-175.

Wagner, T. J. (1985). Smoking behavior of nurses in western New York. *Nursing Research, 34,* 58-60.

Willett, W. C., Browne, M. L., Bain, C., Lipnick, R. J., Stampfer, M. J., Rosner, B., Colditz, G. A., & Hennekens, C. H. (1985). Relative weight and risk of breast cancer among premenopausal women. *American Journal of Epidemiology, 122,* 731-740.*

Willett, W. C., Manson, J. E., Stampfer, M. J., Colditz, G. A., Rosner, B., Speizer, F. E., & Hennekens, C. H. (1995). Weight, weight change, and coronary heart disease in women. *Journal of the American Medical Association, 273,* 461-465.*

Willett, W. C., Stampfer, M. J., Manson, J. E., Colditz, G. A., Rosner, B. A., Speizer, F. E., & Hennekens, C. H. (1996). Coffee consumption and coronary heart disease in women. *Journal of the American Medical Association, 275,* 458-462.*

Woolley, A. S. (1984). Questioning the mailed questionnaire as a valid instrument for research in nursing education. *Image, 16,* 115-119.

STUDY SUGGESTION

Choose one of the articles that reports some of the findings of the Nurses' Health Study and write a short critique (both positive and negative criticism) of that article, paying particular attention to the extent to which the authors attempt to claim causality and/or to generalize the results beyond the population that was actually sampled.

CHAPTER 7

Correlational Research I: "Ordinary" Correlational Studies

CHAPTER OUTLINE

A Taxonomy of Correlational Research
Ordinary Exploratory Correlational Studies
Ordinary Predictive Correlational Studies
Ordinary Explanatory Correlational Studies
Study Suggestions

Key Terms: correlational research, causal-comparative research, prospective (longitudinal) study, cross-sectional study, retrospective study, case-control study, ex post facto research

Correlational research is a catch-all term for studies that examine the relationships between variables. Unlike experiments or quasi-experiments, correlational studies lack active manipulation of the independent variable(s). Therefore, postulation of relationships in causal terms is risky. However, the investigation of associations in correlational studies some-

times gives an indication of how likely it is that a cause-and-effect relationship *might* exist. For example, a report of a strong association between
primary care nursing and expressed client satisfaction with nursing care
may suggest that assignment of clients to a primary nurse is likely to result
in client satisfaction, whereas a weak association between other systems for
providing care and client satisfaction with the care may suggest that clients
are not as likely to express satisfaction with other care modalities.

Despite its limitations, one advantage of the correlational approach is
its applicability to many nursing situations in which experimentation is
impossible or impractical. Questions such as "Does a person's cultural
background affect perception of and response to pain?" are examples in
which the independent variable is a characteristic of an individual that
cannot be manipulated experimentally. Other types of research questions
about the effects of certain treatments on people often cannot be studied
experimentally because of ethical considerations associated with forcing
some clients to receive possibly harmful treatments and/or withholding
possibly beneficial treatments from other clients. There also are instances
in which assignment of subjects to treatment groups is impractical or
beyond the investigator's ability to carry out.

Additional advantages cited in the research literature have to do with
the capacity of correlational designs to deal with large amounts of data
connected with a specific problem area and their strong link to reality in
contrast to the artificiality of laboratory experiments.

A TAXONOMY OF
CORRELATIONAL RESEARCH

What I call "ordinary" correlational studies are those studies that
investigate patterns of relationships between variables by using traditional
correlation coefficients (e.g., Pearson r's [see Chapter 11]). Some are
concerned solely with *exploration;* the strengths and directions of the
relationships are interesting in and of themselves. Others are aimed at
prediction; if the relationship between two variables is strong, then predictions of one variable from the other are likely to be accurate (even though
causality may not be demonstrated). Still others seek an *explanation* of
phenomena that have sound theoretical underpinnings.

What I call **causal-comparative** studies are those studies that compare two or more groups on one or more variables for the purpose of generating causal hypotheses regarding group differences. They are of three types. **Prospective (longitudinal) studies** involve the examination of variables that may produce certain future effects. Studies of this sort tend to require large samples followed over long periods of time. For example, there are ongoing studies to determine whether taking oral contraceptives might be associated with the incidence of stroke or embolism. **Cross-sectional studies** involve the comparison of two or more groups at a single point in time. **Retrospective studies** involve the examination of variables that might have produced certain effects. This approach is common in epidemiological research in which specified diseases may be determined to be associated with prior health conditions or sources of infection. Such studies are called **case-control studies** because "cases" (persons having the disease) are compared to "controls" (persons not having the disease).

I use the term **ex post facto research** as synonymous with retrospective causal-comparative research. Other authors (e.g., Polit & Hungler, 1995) use that term to refer to almost any type of nonexperimental research. I prefer the more restricted meaning to identify experiment-like studies in which the subjects have been exposed to certain "treatments" but were not *assigned* to them. In prospective investigations, group membership is the independent variable and the groups are followed up and measured on one or more dependent variables; in retrospective investigations, group membership is the *dependent* variable and the researcher looks back in time for one or more *independent* variables that may be related to group membership.

Studies concerned with the connection between cigarette smoking and lung cancer are prototypical (by anybody's definition) ex post facto studies. You start with two groups of subjects—those who have lung cancer and those who do not—and carry out a retrospective investigation regarding *whether or not* the various subjects smoked cigarettes, or *how many* cigarettes they smoked, to determine the extent to which cigarette smoking is associated with lung cancer. If there is an association, then it may or may not be causal. In the absence of a controlled experiment, causality would have to be established on other grounds.

This chapter is concerned with ordinary correlational studies. Chapter 8 treats causal-comparative studies (and a couple of studies that have both ordinary and causal-comparative features). Unlike ordinary correlational

Correlational Research

"Ordinary" Correlational Studies   *Causal-Comparative Studies*
Exploratory   Prospective (Longitudinal)
Predictive   Cross-Sectional
Explanatory   Retrospective ("Ex Post Facto")

Figure 7.1. A Taxonomy of Correlational Research

research, causal-comparative studies typically focus on differences between means or quotients of percentages rather than on correlation coefficients.

The diagram in Figure 7.1 may be helpful in clarifying the distinctions made in the preceding paragraphs.

Several nursing research examples of ordinary correlational studies of the exploratory, predictive, and explanatory types are provided in this chapter.

ORDINARY EXPLORATORY CORRELATIONAL STUDIES

A typical example of exploratory correlational research that appeared recently in the nursing literature is the study by Gross, Conrad, Fogg, Willis, and Garvey (1995) of the relationship between mothers' depression and their preschool children's mental health. In the body of the article, several correlation coefficients are reported, not only between the two variables of principal interest but also between each of those variables and other variables such as (children's) social competence. The study was exploratory in that there was no attempt to determine whether or not, or to what extent, one variable is predictable by, or explainable by, another.

Another recent example is the study by Coward (1996) of the various correlates of "self-transcendence." Although the concept of self-transcendence is a theoretical notion, the author was interested not in testing a theory of self-transcendence but merely in exploring the extent to which measures of that concept correlated with other variables.

A third example of exploratory correlational research, one that appeared in the nursing literature a few years ago, is the study by Thomas and Groer (1986) of the relationships between background variables such as age and residence and health-related variables such as stress and blood pressure. The subjects of their investigation were 323 high school freshmen in Tennessee. They were given a test of "life stress"; filled out a questionnaire that asked for information regarding lifestyle (diet, exercise, smoking behavior, etc.) as well as age, sex, and the like; and then had their height, weight, and blood pressure measured. The authors' principal interest was in the simple relationship between the blood pressure readings (diastolic and systolic) and each of the following variables: body mass index, sex, type of residence, age, life stress, amount of exercise, and smoking behavior.

ORDINARY PREDICTIVE CORRELATIONAL STUDIES

Correlational research of the predictive variety is exemplified by the study carried out by Koniak-Griffin and Brecht (1995). They were interested in the extent to which risky behaviors engaged in by adolescent mothers—having multiple sex partners and engaging in unprotected sex—could be predicted by ethnicity, substance abuse, AIDS knowledge, and whether or not the subject was currently pregnant. The findings were mixed; the relative importance of each predictor variable depended on which of the two behaviors was being predicted.

A second example of predictive correlational research is the study by Munro (1985) of graduate clinical specialty programs. She was interested in the extent to which six measures used by the admissions committee at Yale University's School of Nursing correlated, individually and collectively, with graduate grade-point average. Of the six measures (Graduate Record Examination verbal score, Graduate Record Examination quantitative score, undergraduate grade-point average, references rating, interview rating, and applicant essay score), the Graduate Record Examination verbal score and the essay score were found to be the best predictors of overall graduate grade-point average for a sample of 435 entering students.

Prediction of the developmental progress of very low birthweight (VLBW) infants was the focus of a study by Schraeder (1986). A sample of 41 VLBW infants (18 males, 23 females) was followed up from birth to

1 year of age. She found that the best predictors of development at 1 year of age were environmental factors such as emotional responsivity of mother and provision of appropriate play materials.

ORDINARY EXPLANATORY
CORRELATIONAL STUDIES

Two studies that are typical of more theoretically oriented explanatory correlational research were the investigations by Johnson, Ratner, Bottorff, and Hayduk (1993) and Yarcheski, Scoloveno, and Mahon (1994). The first of these was a test of Pender's Health Promotion Model and employed the more complicated technique of structural equation modeling (using the computer program LISREL) in that test. Pender's model was not found to fit the empirical data very well. The second study was a comparison of two path models that might help to explain the effect of perceived social support on general well-being; one model postulated only a direct effect, whereas the other postulated both a direct effect and an indirect effect mediated by hopefulness. Traditional regression analysis was employed in that comparison and the results better supported the model that incorporated the hopefulness variable.

Several older studies dealing with social support also were theoretically oriented. One was the investigation by Norbeck (1985) of job stress in critical care nursing, and another was a similar study of psychological distress among caregivers of the elderly by Baillie, Norbeck, and Barnes (1988). The first of these was a test of LaRocco, House, and French's (1980) model of occupational stress, and the second used House's (1981) stress-buffering model to test the effects of perceived caregiver stress and social support on caregiver distress. The data for a sample of 164 critical care nurses in the first study supported the main effects postulated in the LaRocco et al. model but not the interaction effects. (The terms "main effect" and "interaction effect" are used in correlational research as well as in experimental research but are used in a less causal sense in the former.) The results for the second study were essentially the same, with significant main effects and nonsignificant interaction effects for a sample of 87 caregivers.

The stress-buffering effect of social support also was studied by Brandt (1984), but in her research the dependent variable was maternal discipline of developmentally delayed children from 6 months to 3 years of age. For her convenience sample of 91 mothers, Brandt, unlike Norbeck (1985) and Baillie et al. (1988), found a strong Support × Stress interaction but no main effect of either independent variable taken separately.

Social support was of concern to Hubbard, Muhlenkamp, and Brown (1984) as well. They studied the relationship between individuals' perceived levels of social support and their self-care practices. Their research actually involved two groups of subjects: 97 elderly adults who were attending activities at a senior citizens center and 133 adults (ages 15-77 years) who were attending a health fair. This was *not* a causal-comparative study because the investigators were not interested in comparing the groups to each other; rather, they wanted to see whether the findings from the first study would be replicated in the second study. They found a strong association between high perceived levels of social support and positive health practices in both studies, but the two samples yielded inconsistent results for the authors' secondary hypotheses regarding differences between married and unmarried subjects. For the elderly sample, the married subjects had higher perceived levels of social support and better health practices than did the unmarried sample, but this was not the case for the more heterogeneous general adult sample.

These examples are illustrative, but not exhaustive, of the various types of ordinary correlational studies that are encountered in the quantitative nursing literature. Additional examples are provided in Chapters 10 and 11.

REFERENCES

Baillie, V., Norbeck, J. S., & Barnes, L. A. (1988). Stress, social support, and psychological distress of family caregivers of the elderly. *Nursing Research, 37,* 217-222.

Brandt, P. A. (1984). Stress-buffering effects of social support on maternal discipline. *Nursing Research, 33,* 229-234.

Coward, D. D. (1996). Self-transcendence and correlates in a healthy population. *Nursing Research, 45,* 116-121.

Gross, D., Conrad, B., Fogg, L., Willis, L., & Garvey, C. (1995). A longitudinal study of maternal depression and preschool children's mental health. *Nursing Research, 44,* 96-101.

House, J. S. (1981). *Work stress and social support.* Reading, MA: Addison-Wesley.

Hubbard, P., Muhlenkamp, A. F., & Brown, N. (1984). The relationship between social support and self-care practices. *Nursing Research, 33,* 266-270.

Johnson, J. L., Ratner, P. A., Bottorff, J. L., & Hayduk, L. A. (1993). An exploration of Pender's Health Promotion Model using LISREL. *Nursing Research, 42,* 132-138.

Koniak-Griffin, D., & Brecht, M.-L. (1995). Linkages between sexual risk taking, substance abuse, and AIDS knowledge among pregnant adolescents and young mothers. *Nursing Research, 44,* 340-346.

LaRocco, J. M., House, J. S., & French, J. R. (1980). Social support, occupational stress and health. *Journal of Health and Social Behavior, 21,* 202-218.

Munro, B. H. (1985). Predicting success in graduate clinical specialty programs. *Nursing Research, 34,* 54-57.

Norbeck, J. S. (1985). Types and sources of social support for managing job stress in critical care nursing. *Nursing Research, 34,* 225-230.

Polit, D. F., & Hungler, B. P. (1995). *Nursing research: Principles and methods* (5th ed.). Philadelphia: Lippincott.

Schraeder, B. D. (1986). Developmental progress in very low birth weight infants during the first year of life. *Nursing Research, 35,* 237-242.

Thomas, S. P., & Groer, M. W. (1986). Relationships of demographic, life-style, and stress variables to blood pressure in adolescents. *Nursing Research, 35,* 169-172.

Yarcheski, A., Scoloveno, M. A., & Mahon, N. E. (1994). Social support and well-being in adolescents: The mediating role of hopefulness. *Nursing Research, 43,* 288-292.

STUDY SUGGESTIONS

1. Choose an article in a nursing research journal that reports the results of an experiment and another article in that same journal (not necessarily the same issue or even the same year) that reports the results of a correlational study dealing with the same general topic.

   a. Do you see why the first study is an experiment and the second study is not?
   b. Is causality claimed in the first article? Should it be? Why or why not?
   c. Is causality claimed in the second article? Should it be? Why or why not?

2. Using the taxonomy presented at the beginning of this chapter, how would you classify the second study? Why?

3. If you were to carry out a study of the effect of type of medication on headache pain, would you adopt the experimental approach or the correlational approach? Why?

CHAPTER 8

Correlational Research II: Causal-Comparative Studies

In the previous chapter, the distinction was made between "ordinary" correlational studies and correlational studies that are of the causal-comparative type. This chapter is devoted to a discussion of studies of the latter type and to a few studies that combined both approaches.

By way of a reminder, causal-comparative studies compare two or more groups on one or more variables and may be prospective (longitudinal), cross-sectional, or retrospective (ex post facto). Some examples now follow.

EXAMPLES OF PROSPECTIVE CAUSAL-COMPARATIVE RESEARCH

An example of a study that is a prospective causal-comparative study is the research reported by Jones (1995). She investigated the perceptions of family functioning of four groups of parents: deaf mothers, deaf fathers, hearing mothers, and hearing fathers. One of the interesting findings was that participation in leisure and recreational activities was ranked higher by deaf parents than by hearing parents.

Keefe, Kotzer, Froese-Fretz, and Curtin (1996) compared, longitudinally over the first 4 months of life, a sample of irritable infants to a sample of nonirritable infants and found, among other things, that the irritable infants suffered significantly more disruption in their sleep-wake states.

Another example of a causal-comparative study of the prospective variety (although it was not "billed" that way) is the investigation by Greenleaf (1983) of the labor force participation of female nurses. She contrasted registered nurses ($n = 124$) with elementary school teachers ($n = 157$) and with a composite "other" group of women ($n = 96$) who were in comparable occupations. Greenleaf defined as occupations comparable with nursing those that "(1) [are] sex-segregated with more than 60% women workers; (2) [are] classified as professional, technical workers by the U.S. Census Bureau; and (3) require some form of certified post-high school education" (p. 307). The data were taken from a study carried out by the National Opinion Research Center at the University of Chicago in the 1970s. (In present-day jargon, she carried out a *secondary analysis* [see Chapter 13].) Although she found little or no difference among the three groups in overall labor force participation rates, the married nurses with children were more likely to be in the labor force than were those without children, whereas the opposite was true for the two comparison groups.

Ouellette, MacVicar, and Harlan (1986) compared a group of 24 female athletes to a "control group" of 40 female nonathletes on a number of variables including percentage body fat and menstrual cycle length. It was causal-comparative because it contrasted two groups (the athletes and the nonathletes) on several variables (percentage body fat, menstrual cycle length, etc.) with the intention of generating causal hypotheses concerning why the two groups might differ on those variables. It was prospective because the two groups were followed across time with data collected each month on cycle, flow length, weight, and skinfold thickness. Finally, it is correlational rather than experimental because the independent variable of group membership was not manipulated. We do not *assign* people to be athletes or nonathletes. That is why the term "control group" was enclosed in quotation marks earlier in the paragraph. The principal findings were that there was a significant difference in mean percentage body fat between the athletes (16.5%) and the nonathletes (21.0%) but that there was not a significant difference in mean cycle length.

EXAMPLES OF CROSS-SECTIONAL CAUSAL-COMPARATIVE RESEARCH

An interesting cross-sectional causal-comparative study was carried out by Wineman, Durand, and Steiner (1994). They were concerned with the difference in coping behaviors between 433 subjects with multiple sclerosis and 257 subjects with spinal cord injuries. Although they found no statistically significant differences overall in either emotion-focused coping or problem-focused coping, there was an interaction effect regarding illness uncertainty and appraisal of life with a disability, indicating that vulnerability was a key antecedent variable.

A simpler causal-comparative study reported by McDougall (1994) compared, cross-sectionally, three groups of older adults—young (55 to 64 years), middle (65 to 74 years), and older (75 to 83 years)—with respect to their "metamemory" as measured by the Metamemory in Adulthood Questionnaire. He found no statistically significant differences among those three groups.

An even simpler example is the study by Allan, Mayo, and Michel (1993), who compared a sample of 36 white women to a sample of 31 black women with respect to values regarding body size.

EXAMPLES OF RETROSPECTIVE
CAUSAL-COMPARATIVE RESEARCH

Lowery and Jacobsen (1984) carried out a retrospective causal-comparative study of nursing turnover. They identified 276 nurses who had been hired by a large metropolitan hospital between January 1979 and December 1981 and who had stayed at least 1½ years. At the time of data collection (a couple of years later), it was determined that 92 of the 276 had left (the "leavers") and that the other 184 had remained on the job (the "stayers"). The researchers obtained access to the personnel files of all subjects (they did not mention anything about the potential ethical problems associated with such access) and compared the two groups on a number of variables for which information previously had been obtained. The principal finding was that the leavers had received significantly lower overall job ratings than had the stayers, with interest and motivation being the main reasons for the lower ratings for the leavers.

A retrospective causal-comparative approach to the study of falling behavior was taken by Janken, Reynolds, and Swiech (1986). They compared a sample of 331 patients 60 years of age or older who had fallen during hospitalization to a random sample of 300 patients of the same age range who had not. They used a chart review, sampling 2 days of documentation (admission day for both groups; day before fall for the fall group, random day for the no-fall group), and identified six factors that were significantly related to subsequent fall status: confusion, building in which the patient resided, sleeplessness, mobility of lower extremities, incontinence, and general weakness.

MORE ON CROSS-SECTIONAL
VERSUS LONGITUDINAL STUDIES

Longitudinal correlational studies almost always are to be preferred to cross-sectional studies whenever causality is of interest and the experimental approach is either impossible or impractical. If X at Time 1 is highly correlated with Y at Time 2, then there is at least a temporal basis for the claim that X caused Y (see Chapter 3), whereas if X and Y are obtained at the same time, then it is less likely that X could have caused Y and more likely that another variable, Z, might have caused both X and Y. Longitudinal studies also are more relevant than cross-sectional studies if the research is concerned with development. For example, 3-year-olds today may differ from 4-year-olds today, but the 3-year-olds may not differ as much from themselves when they get to be 4-year-olds.

Longitudinal studies have a number of disadvantages, however. First, they are invariably more costly—in terms of time, money, and effort—than cross-sectional studies. Comparing 50-year-olds, 60-year-olds, and 70-year-olds in the year 2000 would be much easier than starting with 50-year-olds in 2000 and following them up over the next 10 and 20 years until they become 60 (in 2010) and 70 (in 2020).

Second, there is the matter of attrition. Getting a group of subjects to continue to participate in any research project that extends over several years is a real challenge. (The Nurses' Health Study, described elsewhere in this book, is an exception.) Some lose interest, others cannot be contacted, and still others die or are unable to participate. This is, of course, especially true of research on the elderly because their morbidity and mortality rates are understandably higher than those of children or young adults. (For some suggestions for minimizing the attrition problem in longitudinal research, see Given, Keilman, Collins, & Given, 1990.)

But even if there are no "dropouts" at all, there is a third problem. People who are subjects in longitudinal studies often are exposed to the same measurement procedures time after time. Taking the same test more than once can produce unwanted "carryover effects" from one time to the next. The first time people are asked about coping strategies, for example, they may give considered and sincere responses, but on repeated testings with the same instrument, their responses on subsequent occasions may be influenced by what they said the first time (nobody really wants to appear inconsistent), they may get bored with the task, or they may make flippant remarks or be less cooperative in general.

Is there a way in which we can design a study so that we have "the best of both worlds" by capitalizing on the respective advantages of the longitudinal and cross-sectional approaches? The answer is yes, as the following section on the cross-sectional-sequential design attests. Aaronson and Kingry (1988) described other ways of combining longitudinal and cross-sectional approaches, but none can compare with the strength of the cross-sectional-sequential design.

THE CROSS-SECTIONAL-
SEQUENTIAL DESIGN

Before I describe this very powerful design and give some examples, I must introduce some jargon and define some terms that occasionally are used rather loosely in certain types of research. For a more extensive discussion of these terms and of differences between the cross-sectional-sequential design and similar designs, see Achenbach (1978), Kovach and Knapp (1989), and Weekes and Rankin (1988).

The first piece of jargon is the notion of a **cohort**. A cohort is a group of people who share a particular starting point (e.g., birth year). Reference often is made in the literature to the 1946 birth cohort (which was almost $1\frac{1}{2}$ times the size of the 1945 birth cohort) or to the "baby boom" cohorts in general (roughly those people who were born between 1946 and 1964). Another example of a cohort might be all the students who began doctoral study in nursing at a particular university in some specified year, say 1990. Given what we know about students who elect to pursue graduate work in professional disciplines, the members of that cohort are unlikely to all be of the same age; therefore, they would not be members of the same birth cohort.

The term "cohort" sometimes is used as a synonym for "friend," as in "She got along well with her cohorts," but its use in research is more restrictive and requires some connection with a given point in time.

Associated with the concept of a cohort is the term "cohort effect." In developmental research, the investigator often is concerned that a finding might hold only for a particular birth cohort or that differences between two age groups might reflect birth cohort differences rather than differences that may be attributable to age per se. As a matter of fact, the careful developmental researcher tries to distinguish among three types of "effects" (the term "effects" is enclosed in quotation marks for the same reason that the term "control group" was so designated earlier [i.e., the context is nonexperimental]): "age effects," "cohort effects," and "time-of-measurement effects." Age effects are differences between or among age groups that hold regardless of cohort or time of measurement. Cohort effects, as already suggested, are differences that hold regardless of age or time of measurement. Time-of-measurement effects are differences that hold regardless of age or cohort. For example, if a cross-sectional study should reveal differences in attitudes toward abortion in the year 2000 between 20-year-old women and 60-year-old women, then that result might not be a true age effect. Women who will be 20 years old in 2000 were born in 1980, 7 years after the Supreme Court decision that legalized abortion, whereas women who will be 60 years old in 2000 were born in 1940 when abortion was not only illegal but also rare. Therefore, this difference is more likely to be a cohort effect than an age effect. When the women who are 20 years old in 2000 get to be 60 years old in 2040, they may feel exactly the same about abortion as they did when they were 20 years old. There also might be something special about the year 2000 that might contribute to a time-of-measurement effect. If a group of 20-year-olds had been compared to a group of 60-year-olds in 1990, then the results might not have been the same. The trouble with a simple cross-sectional design is that none of this can be sorted out.

But enough of that; now for the design itself. Figure 8.1, adapted from Achenbach (1978), depicts an example of a **cross-sectional-sequential design** that could be used to try to separate out age, cohort, and time-of-measurement effects in cognitive development from 5 to 9 years of age. (Kovach & Knapp, 1989, described a similar design that could be used at the opposite end of the age spectrum.) In this design, three simple random samples (see Chapter 9 for a definition of a simple random sample) are drawn from each of three birth cohorts: children born in 1992, 1993, and 1994. One of the three samples from the 1994 cohort is studied when its members are 5 years old (in 1999), another when *its* members are 6 years old (in 2000), and the third when *its* members are 7 years old (in 2001). Similarly, one of the three samples from the 1993 cohort is studied at 6 years of age (in 1999), another at 7 years of age (in 2000), and the third at 8 years of age (in 2001). To complete the design, the three samples from the 1992 cohort are studied at 7, 8, and 9 years of age, respectively. If all goes well (see the following paragraph for the sorts of things that can be troublesome), then not only can you distinguish among age, cohort, and time-of-measurement effects (because you have data for three cohorts and three times of measurement across the 5-year age span), but you do not have to worry about attrition or carryover effects and you get 5 years worth of developmental information in a 3-year study.

There are a few problems with this design:

Time of Measurement

Cohort	1992			1999	2000	2001
	1993		1999	2000	2001	
	1994	1999	2000	2001		
	5	6	7	8	9	
			Age			

Figure 8.1. A Cross-Sectional-Sequential Design (adapted from Achenbach, 1978)

1. The sample sizes may be too small to be representative of the respective cohorts, and there may be so much sampling error that mistakes in inference are made.

2. The "anchors" may not work; for example, the 6-year-olds in the 1993 cohort may differ from the 6-year-olds in the 1994 cohort so that you cannot use their data interchangeably to follow a developmental path from 5 through 9 years of age (i.e., you cannot jump from the bottom row of Figure 8.1 to the row above it, much less the row above that). This would, of course, be an interesting finding in and of itself because it is indicative of a cohort effect.

3. You have to give up all interest in individual subjects because you do not have data on the same people across time. This turns out to be less of a disadvantage than it might seem, however, because to a "hard-nosed" researcher who espouses the quantitative tradition, each subject is at best a random representative of some population of interest, whereas to a clinician, each subject is a unique human.

Despite these drawbacks, the cross-sectional-sequential design is the best design there is for good, yet feasible, developmental research.

STUDIES THAT ARE BOTH
ORDINARY AND CAUSAL-COMPARATIVE

An interesting article that reports the results of a causal-comparative study that has both ordinary and causal-comparative aspects is that by

Cowan and Murphy (1985), which dealt with the aftermath of the volcanic eruption of Mount St. Helens in 1980. The report concentrated on the initial comparison of two groups of people: 69 bereaved subjects who were family or friends of disaster victims and 50 "controls" who were not directly touched by disaster-related losses. The study on which that report was based is an ordinary correlational study within a causal-comparative study because the authors were primarily interested in the prediction of depression, somatization, and physical health status for each group separately. The independent variables were sex, age, life stress, type of relationship with the deceased, "preventability" of the catastrophic death, and social support.

Murphy (1988) then followed up, 2 years later, 85 (49 bereaved, 36 nonbereaved) of the original 119 subjects to determine whether mental distress in 1981 was a better or worse predictor of mental distress in 1983 than were various background variables, life stress in 1983, and other mediating variables. The results were rather complicated, with one subset of variables found to be the best predictors for one of the two groups and a different subset found to be best for the other group.

Murphy and her colleagues published several other articles based on that same study. The interested reader is referred to Kiger and Murphy (1987), Murphy (1984, 1986a, 1986b, 1987, 1989a, 1989b), and Murphy and Stewart (1985-1986).

Another example of a correlational study that is both ordinary and causal-comparative is the research that was reported by Mercer, Ferketich, and their colleagues in a series of eight articles that were published in *Nursing Research* in the late 1980s and early 1990s (Ferketich & Mercer, 1994, 1995a, 1995b; Mercer & Ferketich, 1990a, 1994a, 1994b; Mercer, Ferketich, DeJoseph, May, & Sollid, 1988; Mercer, May, Ferketich, & DeJoseph, 1986) and three articles that were published in other journals (Mercer & Ferketich, 1990b, 1993, 1995). That study addressed a number of research questions concerning high-risk mothers versus low-risk mothers and "experienced" (multiparous) mothers versus "inexperienced" (primaparous) mothers with respect to a variety of dependent variables such as maternal role competence and maternal-infant attachment. Similar comparisons were made for their partners. That was the causal-comparative aspect for which differences between mean scores were used. The investigators also determined what independent variables were most predictive of those same dependent variables for various subgroups. That was the ordinary correlational aspect, employing Pearson product-moment correlation coefficients and regression analysis (see Chapter 11). Surprisingly, they found very small differences between high-risk and low-risk mothers and their partners and between experienced and inexperienced mothers and their partners.

(You may have noticed that Murphy and her colleagues, as well as Mercer, Ferketich, and their colleagues, published several articles that were actually based on a single study. Whether or not, or under what circumstances, that is appropriate is discussed in Chapter 20.)

A recent study that had both ordinary and causal-comparative features was carried out by Berry, Vitalo, Larson, Patel, and Kim (1996). They were interested in the differences between older men and older women in respiratory muscle strength and also in the correlations between muscle strength and other physical variables *within sex*.

CASE-CONTROL STUDIES

As I pointed out in Chapter 7, in epidemiological research, retrospective causal-comparative studies (i.e., ex post facto studies) are called case-control studies. Such studies are increasingly common in nursing research. A recent example of a case-control study is the research reported by Skoner, Thompson, and Caron (1994). They compared, retrospectively, 94 women with stress urinary incontinence and 46 women without stress urinary incontinence. They identified a number of risk factors that differentiated between the two groups, such as vaginal delivery versus cesarean section, and found that the former contributed the greater risk.

Another example of a case-control study (but not conceptualized as such) is the research carried out by Medoff-Cooper, Delivoria-Papadopoulos, and Brooten (1991), who compared a small sample of five premature infants who had intraventricular hemorrhage to a sample of 25 other premature infants who did not on a number of variables such as mental status, tremulousness, and cerebral metabolism.

An example of the opposite situation, an investigation of substance abuse by nurses that was conceptualized as a case-control study but really is not, was reported by Trinkoff, Eaton, and Anthony (1991). A multistage probability sample of households yielded 143 currently employed registered nurses. Each of those nurses was matched on sex and geographical location with approximately 10 counterparts who were not nurses ($n =$ 1,410) and who were called "controls." All subjects had provided information regarding drug and alcohol abuse in standardized interviews. It was found that the prevalences of illicit drug use of nurses and non-nurses were similar but that the prevalence of alcohol abuse of nurses was smaller. The reason why this study is not a case-control study is that the cases were nurses and the controls were non-nurses, and the emphasis was on the differences between those two groups with respect to drug and alcohol abuse. Nurse/non-nurse is not the dependent variable of interest; abuse/nonabuse is. If the researchers had selected as cases a group of nurses who had abused drugs and/or alcohol and had chosen as controls a group of nurses who had not abused drugs or alcohol with an attempt to identify variables prior to abuse that might be predictive of it, then the study would properly fall under the case-control rubric.

If you are interested in further information regarding case-control studies, then see the article by Polivka and Nickel (1992) and the textbook by Schlesselman (1982). For more on epidemiological research in general, see Feinstein (1985), Hennekens and Buring (1987), and Ryan (1983). Feinstein (1985) is a severe critic of case-control studies, denigrating them as "trohoc" ("cohort" spelled backward) studies.

REFERENCES

Aaronson, L. S., & Kingry, M. J. (1988). A mixed method approach for using cross-sectional data for longitudinal inferences. *Nursing Research, 37,* 187-189.

Achenbach, T. M. (1978). *Research in developmental psychology.* New York: Free Press.

Allan, J. D., Mayo, K., & Michel, Y. (1993). Body size values of white and black women. *Research in Nursing & Health, 16,* 323-333.

Berry, J. K., Vitalo, C. A., Larson, J. L., Patel, M., & Kim, M. J. (1996). Respiratory muscle strength in older adults. *Nursing Research, 45,* 154-159.

Cowan, M. E., & Murphy, S. A. (1985). Identification of postdisaster bereavement risk predictors. *Nursing Research, 34,* 71-75.

Feinstein, A. R. (1985). *Clinical epidemiology.* Philadelphia: W. B. Saunders.

Ferketich, S. L., & Mercer, R. T. (1994). Predictors of paternal role competence by risk status. *Nursing Research, 43,* 80-85.

Ferketich, S. L., & Mercer, R. T. (1995a). Paternal-infant attachment of experienced and inexperienced fathers during infancy. *Nursing Research, 44,* 31-37.

Ferketich, S. L., & Mercer, R. T. (1995b). Predictors of role competence for experienced and inexperienced fathers. *Nursing Research, 44,* 89-95.

Given, B. A., Keilman, L. J., Collins, C., & Given, C. W. (1990). Strategies to minimize attrition in longitudinal studies. *Nursing Research, 39,* 184-186.

Greenleaf, N. P. (1983). Labor force participation among registered nurses and women in comparable occupations. *Nursing Research, 32,* 306-311.

Hennekens, C. H., & Buring, J. E. (1987). *Epidemiology in medicine.* Boston: Little, Brown.

Janken, J. K., Reynolds, B. A., & Swiech, K. (1986). Patient falls in the acute care setting: Identifying risk factors. *Nursing Research, 35,* 215-219.

Jones, E. G. (1995). Deaf and hearing parents' perceptions of family functioning. *Nursing Research, 44,* 102-105.

Keefe, M. R., Kotzer, A. M., Froese-Fretz, A., & Curtin, M. (1996). A longitudinal comparison of irritable and nonirritable infants. *Nursing Research, 45,* 4-9.

Kiger, J., & Murphy, S. A. (1987). Reliability assessment of the SCL-90-R using a longitudinal bereaved disaster population. *Western Journal of Nursing Research, 9,* 572-588.

Kovach, C. R., & Knapp, T. R. (1989). Age, cohort, and time-period confounds in research on aging. *Journal of Gerontological Nursing, 15*(3), 11-15.

Lowery, B. J., & Jacobsen, B. S. (1984). On the consequences of overturning turnover: A study of performance and turnover. *Nursing Research, 33,* 363-367.

McDougall, G. J. (1994). Predictors of metamemory in older adults. *Nursing Research, 43,* 212-218.

Medoff-Cooper, B., Delivoria-Papadopoulos, M., & Brooten, D. (1991). Serial neurobehavioral assessments of preterm infants. *Nursing Research, 40,* 94-97.

Mercer, R. T., & Ferketich, S. L. (1990a). Predictors of family functioning eight months following birth. *Nursing Research, 39,* 76-82.

Mercer, R. T., & Ferketich, S. L. (1990b). Predictors of parental attachment during early parenthood. *Journal of Advanced Nursing, 15,* 268-280.

Mercer, R. T., & Ferketich, S. L. (1993). Predictors of partner relationships during pregnancy and infancy. *Research in Nursing & Health, 16,* 45-56.

Mercer, R. T., & Ferketich, S. L. (1994a). Maternal-infant attachment of experienced and inexperienced mothers during infancy. *Nursing Research, 43,* 344-351.

Mercer, R. T., & Ferketich, S. L. (1994b). Predictors of maternal role competence by risk status. *Nursing Research, 43,* 38-43.

Mercer, R. T., & Ferketich, S. L. (1995). Experienced and inexperienced mothers' maternal competence during infancy. *Research in Nursing & Health, 18,* 333-343.

Mercer, R. T., Ferketich, S. L., DeJoseph, J., May, K. A., & Sollid, D. (1988). Effect of stress on family functioning during pregnancy. *Nursing Research, 37,* 268-275.

Mercer, R. T., May, K. A., Ferketich, S., & DeJoseph, J. (1986). Theoretical models for studying the effects of antepartum stress on the family. *Nursing Research, 39,* 339-346.

Murphy, S. A. (1984). Stress levels and health status of victims of a natural disaster. *Research in Nursing & Health, 7,* 205-215.

Murphy, S. A. (1986a). Perceptions of stress, coping, and recovery one and three years after a natural disaster. *Issues in Mental Health Nursing, 8,* 63-77.

Murphy, S. A. (1986b). Status of natural disaster victims' health and recovery three years later. *Research in Nursing & Health, 8,* 331-340.

Murphy, S. A. (1987). Self-efficacy and social support: Mediators of stress on mental health following a natural disaster. *Western Journal of Nursing Research, 9,* 58-86.

Murphy, S. A. (1988). Mental distress and recovery in a high-risk bereavement sample three years after untimely death. *Nursing Research, 37,* 30-35.

Murphy, S. A. (1989a). An explanatory model of recovery from disaster loss. *Research in Nursing & Health, 12,* 67-76.

Murphy, S. A. (1989b). Multiple triangulation: Applications in a program of nursing research. *Nursing Research, 38,* 294-297.

Murphy, S. A., & Stewart, B. J. (1985-1986). Linked pairs of subjects: A method for increasing the sample size in a study of bereavement. *Omega, 16,* 141-153.

Ouellette, M. D., MacVicar, M. G., & Harlan, J. (1986). Relationship between percent body fat and menstrual patterns in athletes and nonathletes. *Nursing Research, 35,* 330-333.

Polivka, B. J., & Nickel, J. T. (1992). Case-control design: An appropriate strategy for nursing research. *Nursing Research, 41,* 250-253, 380.

Ryan, N. M. (1983). The epidemiological method of building causal inference. *Advances in Nursing Science, 5*(2), 73-81.

Schlesselman, J. J. (1982). *Case-control studies.* New York: Oxford University Press.

Skoner, M. M., Thompson, W. D., & Caron, V. A. (1994). Factors associated with risk of stress urinary incontinence in women. *Nursing Research, 43,* 301-306.

Trinkoff, A. M., Eaton, W. W., & Anthony, J. C. (1991). The prevalence of substance abuse among registered nurses. *Nursing Research, 40,* 172-175.

Weekes, D. P., & Rankin, S. H. (1988). Life-span developmental methods: Application to nursing research. *Nursing Research, 37,* 380-383.

Wineman, N. M., Durand, E. J., & Steiner, R. P. (1994). A comparative analysis of coping behaviors in persons with multiple sclerosis or a spinal cord injury. *Research in Nursing & Health, 17,* 185-194.

STUDY SUGGESTION

See whether you can identify a study in a recent issue of any of the nursing research journals (a study that was not cited in this chapter) that is of the causal-comparative type and write a short critique of that study.

PART C

QUANTITATIVE TECHNIQUES FOR DATA GATHERING AND ANALYSIS

Chapters 9 to 12 are the most technical chapters in the book, dealing with sampling, measurement, statistics, and computers, respectively. Technical does not mean mathematical, however, given that there are no formulas whatsoever. References are made to other sources that do provide the appropriate formulas for those who may be interested.

In Chapter 9, I define the key concepts in sampling, explain the difference between probability sampling and nonprobability sampling, and discuss the crucial matter of sample size.

Chapter 10, on measurement, is the longest chapter in the book. The reason for this is my very strong conviction that measurement is the weakest link in nursing research (and in most other research, for that matter) and that there are many difficult issues that need to be addressed including, but not limited to, various types of validity and reliability. I suggest that you pay close attention to the chapter outline that is provided at the beginning of the chapter so that you do not miss seeing the forest because of all of the trees that are in the way.

Because this is a nursing research text and not a statistics book, in Chapter 11 I try to concentrate on those features of data analysis that are most important in understanding and carrying out the statistical techniques that are most commonly encountered in quantitative nursing research studies. Here, too, you are well advised to attend to the chapter outline.

Chapter 12, on computers, is one of the shortest chapters in the book, not because I think computers are unimportant but rather because researchers' preferences for computers and computer programs are so idiosyncratic. As I point out in that chapter, computers can be used for actual data collection and for the preparation of research reports in addition to their traditional uses for data entry and "massaging."

Sampling

Key Terms: target population, sampled population, drawn sample, responding sample, probability sampling, nonprobability sampling, simple random sampling, stratified random sampling, multistage cluster sampling, sampling frame, census sampling, quota sampling, volunteer sampling, convenience sampling, snowball sampling, purposive sampling, systematic sampling, power analysis

Selecting a part to represent the whole is common in everyday life (e.g., wine tasting) and in social research (e.g., Gallup polls). Yet, with the exception of certain types of surveys, sampling considerations tend to receive short shrift in nursing research. From a scientific point of view, it is hard to imagine anything more important than the representativeness of the sample on which an investigation has been based. What good is it to know, for example, that there is a very strong relationship between two variables, x and y, if that relationship may hold only for the particular sample that just happened to be available at the time?

In this chapter, I explore some basic concepts in sampling, discuss various types of sampling designs and ways of determining sample size, and provide several examples of sampling designs that have been used in recent nursing studies.

BASIC CONCEPTS

The most important terms in sampling are **target population, sampled population, drawn sample**, and **responding sample.** The target population is the population about which the researcher cares. The sampled population is the population that is actually sampled. The drawn sample is the group chosen to be studied. The responding sample is the group that is actually studied. If all goes well (and it usually does not!), then it is possible to generalize the results that are obtained for the responding sample to the results that would be obtained for the target population.

Consider two extreme hypothetical examples. In the first example, the target population is all the Alzheimer's disease patients in the United States; the sampled population is all the Alzheimer's patients at the Veterans Administration Hospital in Buffalo, New York; the drawn sample is a stratified (by age) random sample (see next section for a definition of a stratified random sample) of 50 patients at that hospital; and the responding sample is 25 (out of the 50) patients for whom permission to participate was granted. In the second example, the target population is all the editors of nursing research journals in the United States, which also is the sampled population, the drawn sample, and the responding sample. The first example sounds more "scientific" because it involves four different layers of sampling and some fancy statistical techniques. But that does not necessarily follow. That example actually has two roadblocks to the generalization from responding sample to target population. First, the sampled population might not be representative of the target population. Second, the responding sample might not be representative of the drawn sample (it differs in at least one respect, namely the propensity to participate in a research study), which renders as hazardous even the generalization from responding sample to *sampled* population. The second example may be less interesting, if for no other reason than the fact that the responding sample is very small (about a dozen or so people), but the generalization from responding sample to target population is perfect because they are one and the same.

Most real-world examples fall somewhere in between these two extremes, as the studies cited near the end of this chapter illustrate.

TYPES OF SAMPLING DESIGNS

Research samples are either **probability samples** or **nonprobability samples,** the former usually being the more desirable. In probability sampling, every object in the population of interest has a *known* probability of being drawn into the sample. For **simple random sampling,** a special type of probability sampling, every sample of a given size N has an *equal* probability of being drawn. The selection of a given object also must be independent of the selection of any other object.

There are two other popular types of probability sampling. The first is **stratified random sampling,** in which the population is divided into two or more subpopulations, or "strata," and a probability sample is selected from each "stratum" on an equal, proportional, or disproportional basis. By drawing samples of proportional size, you can ensure that the composite sample is representative of the population with respect to at least one variable, namely the variable (sex, race, etc.) that produced the strata. For a simple random sample without stratification, the sample is only *likely* to be representative. A simple random sample of 25 people drawn from a large population that is 50% male and 50% female could (but probably would not) consist of all same-sex members.

Another type of probability sampling is **multistage cluster sampling.** At the first stage of such a sampling design, 10 large cities might be drawn at random; at the second stage, 2 hospitals might be drawn at random from each of the 10 cities; finally, all nurses at each of those 20 hospitals might be asked to participate in the research. This is different from (and easier than) having a **sampling frame** (population list) of nurses and drawing a simple random sample of nurses from that sampling frame (you need only the lists of cities and hospitals). The analysis of the data for the former case also is different (and more complicated) because between-hospital and between-city variation must be taken into account as well as between-nurse variation.

A "degenerate" type of probability sampling is **census sampling.** Here the entire population is sampled; that is, each object has a probability $= 1$ of being drawn into the sample, and any sort of statistical inference (see Chapter 11) from sample to population is unnecessary.

The term "nonprobability sampling" includes all sampling procedures in which chance plays no role in the determination of the actual constitution of the sample. Some of these are as follows:

1. **Quota sampling.** This resembles stratified random sampling, but instead of stratifying a population on a variable such as sex and taking a simple random sample of, say, 100 men from the male stratum and 100 women from the female stratum, the researcher selects *any* 100 men and *any* 100 women from the population.

2. **Volunteer sampling.** The researcher places an ad in the newspaper, posts a sign-up sheet (or whatever), and carries out a study based on those people who happen to show up.

3. **Convenience ("grab") sampling.** This is volunteer sampling without a notice; that is, the researcher selects as subjects any readily available people (or mice or whatever the appropriate units are). Convenience sampling is, far and away, the most common type of sampling employed in nursing research.

4. **Snowball sampling.** This is a rather strange procedure in which the researcher obtains the initial cooperation of a few subjects, each of them asks other subjects to participate, and so on, until the desired sample size is reached.

5. **Purposive sampling.** This is just what it sounds like. The researcher selects certain individuals having prespecified characteristics who are likely to contribute better than are other individuals to the specific purpose(s) of the study. Sampling continues until it is felt that additional subjects would be unnecessary.

One type of sampling that could fall under either heading is **systematic sampling,** that is, sampling of every k^{th} object. If the starting point in sampling from a list is chosen at random, then there is a probabilistic aspect. If not, then that type of sampling falls into the nonprobability category. See Floyd (1993) for a thorough discussion of systematic sampling.

Figure 9.1 attempts to summarize the various types of probability and nonprobability designs in the context of the four basic sampling concepts. For more specific details regarding these and other sampling designs, see

Target Population
Sampled Population
Drawn Sample
Responding Sample

Probability Sampling	*Nonprobability Sampling*
— simple random sampling	— quota sampling
— stratified random sampling	— volunteer sampling
— multistage cluster sampling	— convenience sampling
— census sampling	— snowball sampling
	— purposive sampling
— systematic sampling	— systematic sampling
(with a random start)	(without a random start)

Figure 9.1. Basic Concepts and Types of Sampling Designs

the book chapter by Giovannetti (1981) and the superb little book by Stuart (1984).

SAMPLE SIZE

The question most often asked of statisticians by researchers is the following: "What size sample should I draw?" The statistician usually answers that question with another question: "How far wrong can you afford to be when you make a sample-to-population inference?" That is the guiding principle in sample size determination. If you cannot afford to be wrong at all, then you must sample the entire population. If you can afford to be "way off," then a very small sample will suffice. There is one exception to this principle. If the population is known to be, or is assumed to be, perfectly homogeneous with respect to the variable(s) in which you are interested, then an N of 1 (any 1) is all you will need.

But when it comes down to actually specifying a particular sample size, you have essentially three choices:

1. Pick an N based solely on practical considerations such as cost and time. If you only have enough money and time to study 10 people, for example, then N is 10.

2. Pick an *N* based on some "rule of thumb" suggested in the methodological research literature (see Chapter 16). One very popular rule, suggested by Nunnally and Bernstein (1994) and many others, is to have at least 10 times as many subjects as you have variables. According to this rule, a simple two-variable correlational study should have *N* equal to or greater than 20, a more complicated 20-variable study should have *N* equal to or greater than 200, and so on. (For more on this matter, see Knapp & Campbell-Heider, 1989.)

3. Pick an *N* by using formulas and tables devised by Cobb (1985), Cohen (1988), Kraemer and Thiemann (1987), and others for yielding the optimal sample size for a given study. It is optimal in the sense of being able to actually specify that the probability of making errors associated with sample-to-population inference will be no larger than whatever amount is tolerable. The Cohen (1988) text and the Kraemer and Thiemann (1987) monograph are the principal reference sources for **power analysis,** currently the most popular way of determining sample size. I am of the opinion, however, that power analysis has been overemphasized and often misused in nursing research (see Knapp, 1996b).

EXAMPLES OF SAMPLING DESIGNS
USED IN NURSING RESEARCH STUDIES

One of the "cleanest" examples of a probability sampling design in the nursing research literature is the simple random sampling technique used by Zimmerman and Yeaworth (1986) in their study of the career success of women in nursing. Using a table of random numbers, they drew a sample of 282 names from a list of 1,834 names in the 1980 *Directory of Nurses With Doctoral Degrees* prepared by the American Nurses Association. Their target population and sampled population were the same—the 1,834 people on the list. The drawn sample consisted of the 282 nurses randomly chosen from that list. But alas, as always happens, not all of the 282 nurses returned the mailed questionnaire, and a second mailing was tried. The responding sample ultimately consisted of 194 subjects.

Reference already has been made in the chapter on surveys (Chapter 6) to the study by Wagner (1985) of nurses' smoking behavior. For that study, the target population (unspecified by Wagner but tacitly assumed) was all nurses (or at least all nurses in the United States). The sampled population was 16,125 registered nurses whose names appeared on a mailing list of nurses in western New York State that was provided by the American Lung Association. The drawn sample was 5% of those nurses ($N = 806$). The responding sample, after three mailings and some telephone calls, was 504 (out of the 806) nurses, a response rate of about 62%. Wagner used a simple random sampling design; the directory provided the sampling frame from which he chose 5% of the names at random. He gave no rationale for the 5%, but it apparently was based on practical considerations.

Keller and Bzdek (1986) used the volunteer approach in their study of therapeutic touch. They recruited subjects from the student health clinic at a particular university, the university's general student and staff population, and the public at large using a combination of radio, newspaper, and bulletin board announcements. Therefore, their target population was people in general (assumed), their sampled population was all the people at that university and its environs, and the drawn sample and responding sample were the same—60 volunteers. (No rationale was provided for an N of 60.)

Although they used a typical convenience sample of readily available patients for their study of patient management of pain medication, King, Norsen, Robertson, and Hicks (1987) were commendably thorough in pointing out just how many subjects participated in the various phases of their study. (A total of 104 patients were asked to participate; of these, 17 refused [the authors even told why], 24 were dropped during the course of the study [the authors also gave the various reasons for that], data were missing for 6 subjects, etc.) The target population is assumed to be all patients, the sampled population was all the patients at the hospital with which the researchers were affiliated, the drawn sample was the 104 originally contacted, and the responding sample varied depending on the particular phase of the study (approximately 50-60 at each phase).

Gulick's (1987) study of the Activities of Daily Living (ADL) Self-Care Scale employed a stratified random sampling design and used Nunnally and Bernstein's (1994) 10-to-1 rule for determining sample size. She drew one third of her sample from a list of approximately 800 members of one of the chapters of the National Multiple Sclerosis Society and two thirds from a second list of approximately 1,600 members of another chapter of that society so that her sample would be proportionately representative of those two populations. The target population undoubtedly is all victims of multiple sclerosis, the sampled population is all the people whose names were on those two lists, the drawn sample consisted of 685 subjects (the scale has 60 items [the variables that were of interest], and 85 "extra" subjects were selected to allow for attrition), and the responding sample was 629 of the 685 (634 agreed to participate, but only 629 completed the ADL Self-Care Scale that was mailed to them) for a response rate of about 92%.

A different sort of sampling design was chosen by Markowitz, Pearson, Kay, and Loewenstein (1981) for their study of knowledge of the hazards of medications on the part of nurses, physicians, and pharmacists. They drew a stratified random sample of 100 registered nurses and a stratified random sample of 102 physicians but selected the entire available population of 14 pharmacists.

Another "mixed-bag" example is provided by the study carried out by Gurklis and Menke (1988) on hemodialysis patients. They used Cohen's tables to determine the drawn (and responding) sample size of 68. The sampling design, however, was one of convenience. The (unspecified) target population is assumed to be all hemodialysis patients, and the sampled population was the group of patients available to the researchers at two outpatient centers in a midwestern city.

An example of one of the most creative types of convenience sampling designs is the technique used by Murphy (1988) in her study of bereavement following the Mount St. Helens eruption in 1980. The sampling plan was carefully described in an article by Murphy and Stewart (1985-1986), but the features bear repeating here. The procedure involved the "linking" of *pairs* of people (one a family member, the other a close friend) to each of the disaster victims in an attempt to increase the size of the sample of bereaved survivors. For the 51 victims identified as confirmed dead or presumed dead, therefore, there was a desired sample size of 102 bereaved friends and relatives. The problem with this sampling plan, however, was the potential lack of "independence of the observations" (a necessary assumption for all statistical tests) because the responses by any linked pair to the questions asked by the researcher (she used mailed questionnaires) might be more similar to one another than each of them would be to the responses of other members of the sample by virtue of the fact that they were concerned with the same victim. In their article, Murphy and Stewart (1985-1986) provided evidence that there appeared to be little *empirical* basis for the dependence of the paired data even though the responses of the pair members were *conceptually* dependent on one another. The sampling plan actually unraveled, as it turned out, because the response rate was such that only 28 of the possible 51 pairs of subjects chose to participate, plus 13 other "halves" of pairs, yielding a total sample size of 69 people who were the bereaved relatives or friends of 41 of the victims. The target population in the Murphy study was all the bereaved survivors of the disaster, the sampled population was all the linked pairs (which also constituted the drawn sample because she tried to get all of them), and the responding sample was the group of 69 who returned the completed questionnaires.

All the foregoing examples are a bit "dated," although they are prototypical illustrations of a variety of sampling plans. For a more recent example, consider the study by Vortherms, Ryan, and Ward (1992). They drew a systematic random sample of 1,173 registered nurses from a population of 43,000 nurses licensed in the state of Wisconsin (responding sample: $N = 790$) for their study of management of cancer pain. Other more recent examples are the simple random sampling plan used by Reed (1992) in drawing a sample of 396 nurses for her study of their provision of emotional care for women who had miscarried and the stratified, multistage random sampling plan chosen by Blegen et al. (1993) in a study of nurses' preferences for decision-making autonomy.

Miller and Champion (1996) studied self-reported mammography use by older women. Although the sample was a convenience sample, it was very large ($N = 1,083$) and quite representative of the target population (women in the United States who are 50 years of age or older) with respect to most of the important demographic variables such as age, years of education, race, income, marital status, and occupational status.

In an article published in that same year, Golding (1996) selected a multistage cluster sample of 6,024 subjects who provided data concerning sexual assaults and the effect they had on physical functioning.

A FEW "CRAFT-TYPE" COMMENTS REGARDING SAMPLING

I would like to close this chapter with some practical advice regarding sample selection. First, start by thinking big. Define the target population that you are really interested in and make some assumptions about its homogeneity with respect to the variables you will be analyzing. If the target population is inaccessible, then you will have to specify some other population as the population to be sampled and you will have to start worrying about the comparability of the sampled and target populations. If the sampled population contains N members and N is not too large, then you may want to sample all of them (if you assume that the population is very heterogeneous) or you may be able to get away with sampling very few of them (if you asume that the population is very homogeneous).

Next, choose a sampling design, ideally some sort of probability sampling. If you are really fortunate and have an actual list of the members of the population, then assign a serial number from 1 to N to each member and use a table of random numbers (they are found in the backs of most statistics textbooks) to draw either a simple random sample or a stratified random sample. Keep in mind that although probability sampling of the sampled population permits generalizability from the drawn sample to the sampled population, such a generalization still is subject to sampling error and the smaller the sample, the larger the error.

Next, evaluate your resources so far as sample size is concerned. If you have a low-budget operation with all sorts of time and money constraints, then decide how many subjects you can handle and draw that number. Only if you can afford the luxury should you start worrying about so many subjects per variable or statistical power. (An exception: If the number of subjects is less than or equal to the number of variables, then you will be in deep trouble when it comes time for data analysis if you do not worry about such things!)

Finally, try very hard to get all the subjects that are drawn to actually participate in the study. If that necessitates extensive following up, cajoling, and the like, then so be it. Remember, the inference you will want to make is from the responding sample to the target population, and if you have a poor response rate, then you cannot even make a defensible inference to the drawn sample, much less to the sampled population or the target population.

REFERENCES

Blegen, M. A., Goode, C., Johnson, M., Mass, M., Chen, L., & Moorhead, S. (1993). Preferences for decision-making autonomy. *Image, 25,* 339-344.
Cobb, E. B. (1985). Planning research studies: An alternative to power analysis. *Nursing Research, 34,* 386-388.

Cohen, J. (1988). *Statistical power analysis for the behavioral sciences* (2nd ed.). Hillsdale, NJ: Lawrence Erlbaum.

Floyd, J. A. (1993). Systematic sampling: Theory and clinical methods. *Nursing Research, 42,* 290-293.

Giovannetti, P. (1981). Sampling techniques. In Y. M. Williamson (Ed.), *Research methodology and its application to nursing* (pp. 169-190). New York: John Wiley.

Golding, J. M. (1996). Sexual assault history and limitations in physical functioning in two general population samples. *Research in Nursing & Health, 19,* 33-44.

Gulick, E. E. (1987). Parsimony and model confirmation of the ADL Self-Care Scale for multiple sclerosis persons. *Nursing Research, 36,* 278-283.

Gurklis, J. A., & Menke, E. M. (1988). Identification of stressors and use of coping methods in chronic hemodialysis patients. *Nursing Research, 37,* 236-239, 248.

Keller, E., & Bzdek, V. M. (1986). Effects of therapeutic touch on tension headache pain. *Nursing Research, 35,* 101-106.

King, K. B., Norsen, L. H., Robertson, K. R., & Hicks, G. L. (1987). Patient management of pain medication after cardiac surgery. *Nursing Research, 36,* 145-150.

Knapp, T. R. (1996b). The overemphasis on power analysis. *Nursing Research, 45,* 379-381.

Knapp, T. R., & Campbell-Heider, N. (1989). Numbers of observations and variables in multivariate analyses. *Western Journal of Nursing Research, 11,* 634-641.

Kraemer, H. C., & Thiemann, S. (1987). *How many subjects?* Newbury Park, CA: Sage.

Markowitz, J. S., Pearson, G., Kay, B. G., & Loewenstein, R. (1981). Nurses, physicians, and pharmacists: Their knowledge of hazards of medications. *Nursing Research, 30,* 366-370.

Miller, A. M., & Champion, V. L. (1996). Mammography in older women: One-time and three-year adherence to guidelines. *Nursing Research, 45,* 239-245.

Murphy, S. A. (1988). Mental distress and recovery in a high-risk bereavement sample three years after untimely death. *Nursing Research, 37,* 30-35.

Murphy, S. A., & Stewart, B. J. (1985-1986). Linked pairs of subjects: A method for increasing the sample size in a study of bereavement. *Omega, 16,* 141-153.

Nunnally, J. C., & Bernstein, I. H. (1994). *Psychometric theory* (3rd ed.). New York: McGraw-Hill.

Reed, K. S. (1992). The effect of gestational age and pregnancy planning status on obstetrical nurses' perceptions of giving emotional care to women experiencing miscarriage. *Image, 24,* 107-110.

Stuart, A. (1984). *The ideas of sampling* (3rd ed.). London: Griffin.

Vortherms, R., Ryan, P., & Ward, S. (1992). Knowledge of, attitudes toward, and barriers to pharmacologic management of cancer pain in a statewide random sample of nurses. *Research in Nursing & Health, 15,* 459-466.

Wagner, T. J. (1985). Smoking behavior of nurses in western New York. *Nursing Research, 34,* 58-60.

Zimmerman, L., & Yeaworth, R. (1986). Factors influencing career success in nursing. *Research in Nursing & Health, 9,* 179-185.

STUDY SUGGESTION

Choose any article from any nursing research journal and identify the following:

1. The target population
2. The sampled population
3. The drawn sample
4. The responding sample
5. The type of sampling
6. The sample size (and how it was determined)

Then write a brief critique of the sampling strategy that was employed, concentrating on some of its weaknesses, if any, and how it could have been improved.

Measurement

Key Terms: measurement, construct, variable, true score, obtained score, validity, reliability, content validity, criterion-related validity, construct validity, sensitivity, specificity, test-retest reliability, parallel-forms reliability, split halves, Cronbach's alpha (coefficient alpha), Guttman scale, interrater reliability, attenuation, nominal scale, ordinal scale, interval scale, ratio scale, semantic differential, Likert-type scale, Q sort

One of the most difficult aspects of research is the "operationalization" of abstractions into concrete terms. Theoretical notions such as pain, stress, and coping need to be articulated in very specific language so that researchers can communicate the results of their studies to interested colleagues and to the subjects of their investigations. Failure to do so could result in vague generalities that have no meaning. However, this is not to say, for example, that *all* pain researchers must define pain in the same way. It just argues for *each* researcher's being responsible for clarifying how pain (or whatever) is to be addressed in any given study.

The process of operationalizing abstract "constructs" into concrete "variables" is called **measurement**. (There are other definitions of measurement [see, e.g., Waltz, Strickland, & Lenz, 1991], but I prefer the operationalization definition.) The first sections of this chapter treat some of the notions that are fundamental to all scientific measurement such as validity and reliability, levels of measurement, and the implications of measurement properties for data analysis. The latter sections treat various types of instruments that are used in quantitative nursing research.

CONSTRUCTS, VARIABLES, TRUE SCORES, AND OBTAINED SCORES

An important distinction that must be made at the outset is the difference between latent characteristics and manifest characteristics. Latent characteristics are the theoretical **constructs** that are of principal scientific interest, whereas manifest characteristics are their operationalizations and are called **variables**. The researcher determines, for any given study, how each of the constructs is to be measured. The measurements that would be produced if the measuring instrument were error free are called **true scores**. (The word "scores" is used here in its most general sense; the measurements may have nothing whatsoever to do with the types of scores that typically are associated with educational testing.) The measurements that are actually produced are called **obtained scores**.

For example, body temperature is a construct (latent characteristic). One operationalization (manifest characteristic) of temperature might be the reading on a particular oral thermometer. The reading that a given person *should* get is that person's true score on the variable. The reading that the person *does* get, which may differ from the true score for any

Table 10.1   Examples of Constructs, Variables, True Scores, and Obtained
Scores

Construct	1. Anatomical knowledge
	2. Height
Variable	1. Percentage of body bones that a person identifies correctly when shown a skeleton
	2. Number of inches from the floor to the top of the head as indicated by the Smith tape measure when a person stands against it
True score	1. Percentage of *all* the body bones that a person *can* identify correctly
	2. Number of inches that the tape measure *should* indicate
Obtained score	1. Percentage of a random sample of 30 bones that a person *does* identify correctly
	2. Number of inches that the tape measure *does* indicate

SOURCE: Adapted from Knapp (1985).

number of reasons (e.g., if the reading was taken on an unusually hot day),
is the obtained score.

Table 10.1, adapted from Knapp (1985), provides two other examples
that illustrate the terms "construct," "variable," "true score," and
"obtained score."

It occasionally happens that a researcher goes from variable to construct rather than from construct to variable; that is, instead of starting
with one or more constructs and operationalizing it (them), a technique
called **factor analysis** is used to generate the number and nature of
underlying constructs from a collection of manifest characteristics whose
latent counterparts are unknown but are of considerable interest. For a
general discussion of factor analysis, both "exploratory" and "confirmatory," see Munro (1997) and Nunnally and Bernstein (1994). In their
exploratory factor analysis, Mahon, Yarcheski, and Yarcheski (1995) found
that a two-factor solution best represented the dimensionality of the
20-item revised UCLA Loneliness Scale for Adolescents. Lowe, Walker, and
MacCallum (1991) carried out a confirmatory factor analysis of the
hypothesized dimensionality of the McGill Pain Questionnaire. (For other
recent examples of factor analyses, see Fawcett & Knauth, 1996, and
Wineman, Durand, & McCulloch, 1994.) The factor-analytic approach to

measurement is particularly appealing in theory construction whereby an attempt is made to reduce the dimensionality of a problem by converting a relatively large number of concrete variables into a relatively small number of abstract constructs that might provide a more parsimonious explanation of a phenomenon.

Think of constructs as fuzzy notions that scientists would like to be able to communicate about but have a great deal of difficulty in doing so. They need to be more down-to-earth regarding constructs such as pain, so they talk about variables such as score on the McGill Pain Questionnaire instead. That instrument produces obtained scores (the scores people *do* get), not the associated true scores (the scores people *should* get).

VALIDITY

"What Does the NCATS Measure?" is the title of an article by Gross, Conrad, Fogg, Willis, and Garvey (1993). That is an example of a research question that asks about the validity of a measuring instrument, in this case the Nursing Child Assessment Teaching Scale.

Validity is a matter of the "fit" between the construct that you are trying to measure and the true score on the corresponding variable. A measuring instrument is valid if a person's true score provides a good indication of the score that would be determined on the construct if the construct were manifest rather than latent. A low reading on a particular thermometer is valid, for example, if the body temperature of the person being measured is "really" cold.

The methodological literature is replete with all types of validity, but the "bottom line" invariably is the agreement among experts that a particular instrument either does or does not properly operationalize the construct of interest.

Approximately every 10 years, a joint committee of the American Psychological Association, the American Educational Research Association, and the National Council on Measurement in Education publishes "Standards" for validity and reliability. (The disciplines of education and psychology historically have paid the most attention to issues regarding validity and reliability.) The first few "Standards" for validity emphasized three types of validity (content, criterion related, and construct), and a discussion of each of those now follows. In the most recent document, however, both content validity and criterion-related validity have been subsumed under construct validity. Two other types of validity, *internal validity* and *external validity,* are properties of research designs, not properties of measuring instruments (see Chapter 5).

CONTENT VALIDITY

To determine whether or not, or to what extent, a given instrument possesses **content validity**, one or more persons who are experts in the discipline in which the instrument is to be employed scrutinize the instrument very carefully and make a value judgment regarding how well the instrument operationalizes the construct it is alleged to measure. Such scrutiny may involve some empirical data, but often it does not. For example, in assessing the validity of a particular questionnaire designed to measure attitudes toward abortion, the person who devises the instrument might ask several experts for their opinions regarding the relevance of each of the items on the questionnaire and may decide to retain an item only if, say, at least 80% of the experts judge it to be an appropriate indicator of the construct. Or, a very large pool of items might be constructed based on statements made by pro-choice and right-to-life forces (say, 200 items of each), with a random sample of 50 items drawn from that pool making up the actual test.

A special subtype of content validity is **face validity**. Here the "experts" are those who are actually being measured with the instrument. If it seems to the test takers that the items on a questionnaire measuring attitudes toward abortion do in fact properly measure such attitudes, then the questionnaire is said to be face valid whether or not the abortion researchers think it is valid. (Some authors define face validity somewhat differently from this, but this is the distinction that I personally prefer.)

An interesting example of a study of face validity that actually involved data provided by potential test takers is the research reported by Beyer and Aradine (1986). In that investigation of the content validity of the "Oucher" (an instrument for measuring pediatric pain), the authors attempted to determine whether children put the pictures of a baby thought to be in various degrees of pain intensity in the same rank order in which the pictures had been sequenced in the original development of the scale. (They actually agreed quite well.)

For a good discussion of the difference between content validity in general and face validity in particular, see Lynn (1986). That article also discussed various ways of quantifying content validity. Some have suggested that certain methods of qualitative research also can be used to help determine content validity (Tilden, Nelson, & May, 1990). An excellent discussion of the treatment of content validity in the nursing research literature as compared to its treatment in the educational and psychological research literature was provided by Berk (1990). For further discussions of face validity, see Nevo (1985), the comment regarding Nevo's article by Secolsky (1987), and the article by Thomas, Hathaway, and Arheart (1992).

I also include under content validity practical matters such as whether or not the test is too long, too invasive, or inappropriate for a given age level. Other authors use terms such as *feasibility* or *practicability* to refer to these matters. Expert judgment regarding such matters is just as important as expert judgment regarding the specific content of the test itself. When preparing an other-language version of a measuring instrument, content validity in the form of "back-translation" is absolutely crucial (see, e.g., Jones, 1987, and Walker, Kerr, Pender, & Sechrist, 1990).

CRITERION-RELATED VALIDITY

To determine the **criterion-related validity** of a measuring instrument, you must compare scores obtained on that instrument to scores for the same persons produced by a highly regarded external instrument that sometimes is called a "gold standard." Such a comparison usually involves some sort of statistical correlation coefficient (see Chapter 11). If the correlation is high, then the instrument whose validity is in question is declared to be valid; if the correlation is low, then its validity is suspect. For example, if you wanted to study the criterion-related validity of a new electronic thermometer, then you could take the temperatures of a random sample of people with the new thermometer and also with a well-established mercury-in-glass thermometer (a gold standard). If each person in the sample has readings on the two thermometers that are very close to one another, then you could claim that the electronic device is valid.

This type of validity is thought to be very important by the scientific community. What could be stronger evidence for the validity of a measuring instrument? But there is a catch. How do we know that the well-established mercury-in-glass thermometer is valid? Is it because its readings correlate highly with some other mercury-in-glass thermometer? How do we know that *that* thermometer is valid? Either we have an infinite series of gold standard comparisons to make or (more likely) one of these has to be taken as *the* criterion on the basis of some sort of expert judgment (i.e., content validity). Whenever the respective roles of predictor and criterion *are* clear, such as when there exists a measure of core temperature (Byra-Cook, Dracup, & Lazik, 1990; Heidenreich & Giuffre, 1990; Heidenreich, Giuffre, & Doorley, 1992), the ambiguity inherent in criterion-related validity often disappears.

Some measurement textbooks discuss two subtypes of criterion-related validity, namely **concurrent validity** and **predictive validity**. The only difference between the two is that for concurrent validity the gold standard measures are obtained at approximately the same time as the scores on the instrument whose validity is under investigation, whereas for predictive validity the gold standard measures are obtained at a future time. The temperature example just described is a good example of concurrent validity. Aptitude tests provide the best examples of predictive validity. A test of nursing aptitude, for example, is said to be valid if people who score high on the test also score high on a test of nursing achievement administered at a later date (perhaps several years later) and if people who score low on the aptitude test score low on the achievement test.

In developing a now well-known measure of social support, Norbeck, Lindsey, and Carrieri (1981, 1983) carried out a number of validity studies of their instrument. In one of their criterion-related validity studies, they used the Social Support Questionnaire of Cohen and Lazarus as the gold standard. They found a variety of correlations between the Norbeck et al. scales and the three Cohen and Lazarus scales (ranging from –.44 to .56) for a sample of 42 first-year graduate students in nursing. It was concurrent validity because the Norbeck et al. and Cohen and Lazarus instruments both were administered to that sample of nurses on the same occasion. (For more on the measurement of social support, see Weinert & Tilden, 1990.)

One question that often is asked is the following: If you have access to a gold standard that can serve as the external criterion for a validity study, then why not use *it* in your research rather than the instrument whose validity is unknown? That is a very good question. The only rationale for not doing so is some sort of "substitutive validity" argument. The gold standard may be too expensive or too complicated (or whatever), and the researcher may be willing to forgo more direct validity to cut costs. Again we turn to temperature measurement for an example. It is possible to use a very expensive, very invasive device to measure core temperature (*the gold standard*), but the decision usually is made to estimate core temperature by oral, rectal, axillary, and/or tympanic measurement with thermometers that are much less expensive and much less invasive.

CONSTRUCT VALIDITY

Construct validity is held in even higher esteem than criterion-related validity by most researchers but is subject to some serious logical and logistical problems. It usually is addressed by hypothesizing certain types of relationships that should hold if the instrument is valid and then investigating the extent to which the hypothesized relationships are supported by empirical evidence. One very popular way in which to study construct validity is the method suggested by Campbell and Fiske (1959). They argued that a valid test of a construct such as pain should correlate higher with other operationalizations of pain (**convergent validity**) than with operationalizations of constructs with which pain might be confused such as fear and anxiety (**discriminant validity**, sometimes called **divergent validity**). To find out whether or not such is the case, you would administer to the same group of people the pain instrument of unknown validity along with at least one other pain instrument that also is of unknown validity; that is, it is *not* a gold standard because if it were, then the type of validity under consideration would be criterion-related validity, not construct validity. You also would administer at least one instrument that alleges to measure something other than pain (e.g., fear). The scores obtained on all three (or more) instruments would then be compared (correlated). The ideal result would be high correlations between the two alleged pain instruments (the convergent aspect) and low, or at least *lower,* correlations between each of the alleged pain measures and the alleged fear measure (the discriminant aspect). Ryan-Wenger (1990) applied the Campbell and Fiske (1959) method to the investigation of the construct validity of the Schoolagers' Coping Strategies Inventory.

But even if the ideal result were to be realized, you would find yourself on the horns of a dilemma. All you would really know is that the two alleged pain measures were converging on the *same* construct (which may or may not be pain) and were diverging from some other construct (which may or may not be fear). There must be an accompanying "act of faith" that the

Construct A

Operationalization a_1

Operationalization a_2

Construct B   Operationalization b

The correlation between a_1 and a_2 is high.
The correlation between a_1 and b is low.
The correlation between a_2 and b is low.
Therefore, a_1 and a_2 appear to be measuring the same thing.
But is it Construct A?
Likewise, b appears to be measuring something different from whatever
          it is that a_1 and a_2 are measuring.
But is it Construct B?

Figure 10.1. The Construct Validity Dilemma

scientists who constructed the two alleged measures of pain cannot both be wrong. (Here we are back to content validity again.) Figure 10.1 depicts the dilemma.

Beyer and Aradine (1988) were concerned with that very problem. They administered three alleged pain measures (the "Oucher" and two others) and two alleged fear measures to a sample of 74 hospitalized children and found that the alleged pain measures correlated highly with one another, the alleged fear measures correlated moderately with one another, and the pain-fear correlations were very small. Therefore, that study provided some empirical evidence for the construct validity of all five measuring instruments.

For a construct validity study of the problem of discriminating between pain and anxiety, see Shacham and Daut (1981). For general discussions of the validity of instruments for measuring pain, see Beyer and Knapp (1986), McGuire (1984), and Puntillo and Weiss (1994). For an extended discussion of the issue of construct validity in the measurement of stress and strain, see Knapp (1988). For an example of a study that investigated the validity and reliability of one measure of the latter (the Parent Caregiver Strain Questionnaire), see England and Roberts (1996).

Factor analysis also plays a role in the determination of construct validity. If, for example, a construct is known to have, or is hypothesized to have, four dimensions but a factor analysis suggests one or six dimensions, then there is an obvious problem of lack of agreement between theory and data.

THE "KNOWN-GROUPS" TECHNIQUE

This is a fairly common procedure for determining the validity of a measuring instrument. In the development of an operationalization of some construct X (where X is pain, stress, coping, or whatever), it would be nice if those people who are alleged to have a lot of X got quite different scores on the operationalization of X than did those people who are alleged to have only a little of X. For example, the validity of a measure of stress would be enhanced if nurses who are single parents scored higher than did single nurses without family responsibilities, assuming that high scores are indicative of more stress and that single parents are more stressed. In most of the nursing literature, such studies are said to fall under the heading of construct validity. I disagree. They are criterion-related validity studies because the gold standard is the variable of group membership (single parents vs. single nurses without family responsibilities). For more on this point, see Knapp (1985).

The known-groups technique also can be used to determine the validity of diagnostic screening tests of various sorts (Larson, 1986). Every diagnostic test should be examined for **sensitivity** (the proportion or percentage of those who have the disease who are diagnosed as having the disease) and **specificity** (the proportion or percentage of those who do not have the disease who are diagnosed as not having the disease). The ideal situation would be perfect sensitivity and perfect specificity, but all measuring instruments are fallible, so the best we can do is to try to minimize "false positives" (people who do not have the disease but are diagnosed as having the disease) and "false negatives" (people who have the disease but are diagnosed as not having the disease). In her article, Larson (1986) gave a hypothetical example of some data for a sample of 47 people that provide estimates of the sensitivity, specificity, false positive rate, and false negative rate for a nurse's clinical assessment of whether or not a patient has a urinary tract infection.

Leidy, Abbott, and Fedenko (1997) also investigated the validity, in this same sense of sensitivity, of a dual-mode "actigraph" for measuring functional performance. The actigraph, a watch-like instrument that is worn on the wrist, is not a diagnostic instrument, but the authors were concerned with the extent to which the instrument could produce electronically recorded measurements that successfully discriminate among light, moderate, and heavy physical tasks. It did so for light versus heavy tasks and for light versus moderate tasks but not for moderate versus heavy tasks. They also studied the instrument's "reproducibility" or reliability (see following sections).

RELIABILITY

It is essential to understand that it is the fit between construct and true score, not obtained score, that is relevant for validity despite the fact that both construct and true score are theoretical, not observable, entities. The corresponding fit between true score and obtained score is a matter of **reliability**, as the following sections attempt to explain.

Even if a particular measuring instrument is thought to provide an ideal operationalization of the construct under consideration, scores on that instrument may be subject to chance fluctuations, with the obtained scores being different from the true scores that would be realized if chance played no role in the measurement process. In the temperature example to which I already have alluded, the best thermometer can be "off" on occasion, yielding a reading that is either a little bit higher or a little bit lower than the person's true temperature for that instrument on that occasion. The extent to which obtained scores deviate from true scores is the province of reliability.

Just as is the case for validity, there are several types of reliability; however, for reliability, the bottom line is not expert judgment but rather empirical verification. Life would be simple if reliability also were primarily a matter of expert judgment, that is, if authorities in the field could scrutinize a measuring instrument and evaluate the extent to which obtained scores *should* approximate true scores for the instrument. Unfortunately, such is not the case. Reliability is strictly an empirical phenomenon. Researchers who contemplate using a particular instrument in their studies must either have or get some evidence indicating that the obtained scores *do* approximate the corresponding true scores. But how is that possible given that the true scores always are unknown? That is where measurement theory comes into play. By making a number of assumptions regarding the behavior of obtained scores and true scores, a variety of techniques involving only obtained scores can be used to evaluate the fit between obtained scores and true scores.

The claim was made in the second paragraph of this section that even the most valid instruments can be unreliable. The converse is actually much more common. There are a lot of measuring devices that are highly reliable but are not valid. For example, consider a 50-item test consisting of true-false questions of the form $x + y = z$ (where x, y, and z are replaced by various single-digit numbers such as 2, 5, and 7), which is alleged by its author to measure verbal aptitude. Such a test would be very reliable; people who know how to add single digits will get consistently high scores, and people who do not will get consistently low scores. But as a measure of verbal aptitude, it is virtually worthless (i.e., invalid).

In a previous section of this chapter I pointed out that scientists prefer to talk about, for example, score on the McGill Pain Questionnaire rather than pain. But merely shifting from construct to variable does not take them off the hook. They still need to distinguish between the score on the McGill Pain Questionnaire that a person should have gotten (true score) and the score that the person did get (obtained score). True scores and obtained scores are on the same scale of measurement with the same set of categories. But we never know the true scores, although we worry about them a lot; all we know are the obtained scores. Validity issues come into play whenever we ask the question, "Does the McGill Pain Questionnaire really measure pain?" (Is there a good fit between the construct and its operationalization?), and reliability issues come into play whenever we ask the question, "How consistently does the McGill Pain Questionnaire measure whatever it is that it measures?" (Is there a good fit between the obtained scores and the corresponding true scores?).

Table 10.2, also adapted from Knapp (1985), uses the same examples given in Table 10.1 to illustrate this difference between validity and reliability.

TEST-RETEST RELIABILITY

One technique for estimating reliability is the **test-retest** procedure. Measurements are obtained on the instrument for the same people (or mice

Table 10.2 The Difference Between Validity and Reliability

	Validity	
Construct	→	*True Score*
Anatomical knowledge		Percentage of *all* the body bones that a person *can* identify correctly
Height		Number of inches that the tape measure *should* indicate

	Reliability	
True Score	→	*Obtained Score*
Percentage of *all* the body bones that a person *can* identify correctly		Percentage of a random sample of 30 bones that a person *does* identify correctly
Number of inches that the tape measure *should* indicate		Number of inches that the tape measure *does* indicate

SOURCE: Adapted from Knapp (1985).

or hospitals or whatever the objects of measurement are) on two closely spaced occasions, and the two sets of measurements are compared. They usually are *correlated* with one another (see Chapter 11), but it often is better to use other statistical methods. (Regarding alternative approaches, see Engstrom, 1988; Jacobsen, Tulman, & Lowery, 1991; and Nield & Gocka, 1993.) If there is very little difference between the obtained scores on the first occasion and the obtained scores on the second occasion, then the instrument is said to be reliable because it yields scores that are stable across time. The duration of the time interval between the two occasions is crucial. It must be short enough that the true scores can be assumed to have remained constant so that any differences between the two sets of obtained scores are "the instrument's fault" and do not represent changes in the construct that has been operationalized, but it must not be so short that the agreement between the two sets of obtained scores is artificially high. Many studies in the nursing literature that have been called test-retest reliability studies have employed such long intervals between measurement occasions that it is unrealistic to expect that the corresponding true scores could have remained constant. Those studies are better thought of as investigations of the stability of the constructs rather than the stability of the instruments, in which cases the stability of the instruments still needs to be addressed (Heise, 1969; Knapp, Kimble, & Dunbar, 1998). Using a test-retest correlation coefficient to assess reliability confounds instrument stability with construct stability. A low test-retest correlation, for example, could be indicative of an unreliable measure of an enduring trait, a reliable measure of a fleeting state, or even an unreliable measure of a fleeting state.

Test-retest reliability is especially relevant for single-item tests such as the question "Does it hurt?," which is a simple, but not unreasonable, approach to the measurement of pain. This example also serves to illustrate the importance of the time interval between asking "Does it hurt?" the first time and asking "Does it hurt?" the second time. Let the interval be too long (1 minute might even be too long in some cases), and the phenomenon itself might change, making the instrument (the single-item test) look more unreliable than it probably is. On the other hand, an interviewer would sound pretty silly asking "Does it hurt?" and "Does it hurt?" in rapid succession. The person being asked to respond (even a very young child) might answer "Yes" and "I told you yes!" in equally rapid succession. Reliability is tricky business.

Norbeck et al. (1981) chose a 1-week interval between test and retest for a study of the reliability of their measure of social support using a sample of 67 students in a master's degree program in nursing. They found test-retest coefficients ranging from .85 to .92 for the various scales. (A coefficient of 1.00 would be indicative of perfect stability of the instrument.) They defended the 1-week interval by arguing that it would "reduce the likelihood of tapping true changes in the students' networks as they became acquainted with each other in the program" (p. 267).

Rock, Green, Wise, and Rock (1984) provided an excellent review of the psychometric properties (scoring, validity, reliability, etc.) of a number of other scales for measuring social support and social networks.

In their assessment of the reproducibility of the Ambulatory Monitoring Actigraph, Leidy et al. (1997) used an interval of varying length for each subject with a mean of 2.8 days ($SD = 1.7$). In my judgment, that is too long because the subjects' "true" abilities to perform the tasks could have changed (somewhat or a great deal) between the first and the second tests despite the fact that the tasks themselves remained identical.

PARALLEL-FORMS RELIABILITY

Another approach to the estimation of the reliability of a measuring instrument is the use of **parallel forms** (sometimes called alternate forms or equivalent forms). It is essentially the same as the test-retest procedure; the only difference is that instead of administering the same instrument on the two occasions, one of two comparable forms is administered at Time 1 and the other at Time 2. (Some researchers get a little fancier and administer Form A at Time 1 to half of the people, Form B at Time 1 to the other half, and then the reverse at Time 2. This is an effort to counterbalance any "practice effect" there may be between forms.) For example, for many years there were two forms of the Stanford-Binet Intelligence Test, actually called Form L and Form M rather than Form A and Form B. Investigations of the reliability of that test often involved the administration of both forms to the same children with 1 or 2 days between administrations (true intelligence is unlikely to change much in a couple of days), with the scores on the two forms correlated with one another. The correlations usually were found to be quite high, thus supporting the claim of high reliability (but not necessarily high validity) of that test.

SPLIT-HALVES RELIABILITY

A third way of investigating reliability is a procedure that is appropriate only for multiple-item cognitive or affective tests. It is called the **split-halves** technique and was invented by two British psychologists named Spearman and Brown in the first part of the 20th century. Instead of having two full-length forms administered on two occasions, you have a single form that is administered just once, but in scoring the test you divide the single form into two half tests (ideally at random but more commonly by assigning the odd-numbered items to one of the two halves and the even-numbered items to the other half). Scores on the two half tests are then correlated with one another as in the parallel-forms technique, but because greater consistency is expected between full tests than between half tests, this correlation is "stepped up" by a formula also invented by Spearman and Brown. The resulting number is used to provide an indication of the **internal consistency** of the test. It provides no evidence for the reliability of the instrument in the stability sense, however, because no time passes between Form A and Form B.

An example of a measurement situation in which the split-halves technique might be useful is the estimation of the internal consistency reliability of the test of attitudes toward abortion referred to earlier. A high split-half correlation, stepped up by the Spearman-Brown formula, would indicate a high degree of homogeneity among the items (they "hang together"), which certainly is desirable if you are going to use a single total score on the test to indicate such attitudes.

CRONBACH'S ALPHA (COEFFICIENT ALPHA)

Another type of internal consistency reliability very closely related to split halves is one that goes by the name of **Cronbach's alpha** or coefficient alpha. It involves a formula that was derived by the well-known educational psychologist Lee Cronbach (1951) for assessing the extent to which the items on a test correlate with one another. The higher the intercorrelations between pairs of items, the higher the item-to-item internal consistency of the test, again providing an indication of the test's reliability in the homogeneity sense, not the stability sense. (It turns out that Cronbach's coefficient alpha is the average of all the possible stepped-up split-half reliabilities.) There also are simpler versions of Cronbach's formulas for dichotomously scored items (1 = *right,* 0 = *wrong*), which were actually derived by Kuder and Richardson several years prior to Cronbach's work. Therefore, it is better to think of the alpha formulas as generalizations of Kuder and Richardson's formulas than to think of the Kuder and Richardson formulas as special cases of Cronbach's alpha.

Coefficient alpha is used for more measuring instruments in quantitative nursing research than all the other types of reliability coefficients combined. That does not necessarily mean it is any better; it is just more popular (Knapp, 1991). It would, of course, be just as appropriate for the test of abortion attitudes as is split halves.

GUTTMAN SCALABILITY

The epitome in internal consistency reliability is a situation investigated many years ago by Guttman (1941). An instrument is said to be perfectly internally consistent if the response of each subject to each test item can be predicted by knowing only the total score for that subject. A person with a total score on an aptitude test of 7 out of 10, for example, would have answered the 7 easiest items correctly and missed the 3 hardest items. The extent to which the items on an instrument conform to a perfect **Guttman scale** can be determined by calculating a statistic called the coefficient of reproducibility.

INTERRATER RELIABILITY

The final type of reliability that is discussed in the methodological literature goes by a variety of names, but the most descriptive term is **interrater reliability.** (Interobserver reliability, interjudge reliability, and intercoder reliability are common synonyms.) Here the emphasis is on the agreement between people who *score* the test. The scores (or ratings or whatever) indicated by Person A are compared to the scores indicated by Person B to determine the degree of consistency between two equally competent people who are making the measurements. For example, if two obstetric nurses cannot agree on the Apgar score to be assigned to a newborn baby, then that instrument is not a very reliable indicator of infant viability. High interrater reliability is especially important in observational studies. There also is a variation of the technique, called *intra*rater reliability, where the interest is in the consistency within the *same* rater (e.g., from one reading of an interview protocol to another).

Interrater reliability can be determined in a number of ways (Cohen, 1960; Fox, 1982; Goodwin & Prescott, 1981), but the two most common procedures involve percentage agreement (the simplest method [for a discussion of that method and other methods for nominal variables, see Topf, 1986b]) and the intraclass correlation coefficient (Armstrong, 1981; Spence Laschinger, 1992; Ventura, Hageman, Slakter, & Fox, 1980). Goldsmith (1981) discussed the use of videotape for establishing interrater reliability in observational research. Gross (1991) provided a similar discussion of the validity of observational data obtained by videotaping.

In the first paragraph of this section, the phrase "equally competent" was used when referring to the various raters. The raters must be of equal status whenever you investigate interrater reliability. If one of the raters is a novice and the other is an expert, then a comparison of the two sets of ratings is actually a matter of validity, not reliability.

Although the validity and reliability of the dependent variable are of primary interest in most research studies, the careful investigator also should be concerned about the validity and reliability of the independent variable(s). Padilla (1984) addressed this all too easily ignored problem.

Table 10.3 summarizes the various types of validity and reliability and how they are determined.

Table 10.3 Types of Validity and Reliability

Validity	
1. Content	Usually involves a subjective determination of validity by one or more experts.
2. Criterion related	"Scores" on the instrument whose validity is under consideration are compared to "scores" on an external "gold standard."
3. Construct	Scores on the instrument are correlated with scores on other instruments alleged to measure the same construct (the convergent aspect) and with scores on instruments alleged to measure dissimilar but confusable constructs (the discriminant aspect).

Reliability	
1. Test-retest	The instrument is administered twice to the same subjects, and the Time 1 scores are compared to the Time 2 scores.
2. Parallel forms	Two equivalent forms are administered to the same subjects, and the two sets of scores are correlated.
3. Split halves	The instrument is administered once but is scored in two halves. The halves are correlated, and that correlation is "stepped up" by the Spearman-Brown formula.
4. Cronbach's alpha (coefficient alpha)	The instrument is administered once, and an item analysis is carried out. One of Cronbach's formulas is then used to get an estimate of the reliability.
5. Interrater	The ratings of two (or more) "judges" are compared with one another to determine the degree of agreement in the *scoring* of the instrument.

ATTENUATION

It often is said that a measuring instrument cannot be valid unless it is reliable. That claim has both a conceptual basis and a statistical basis. The conceptual reason why an instrument usually cannot be valid and unreliable is that if the instrument does not produce consistent scores, then it cannot properly operationalize the underlying construct. The statistical reason is embodied in a formula called the "correction for attenuation" formula (Abraham, 1994; Muchinsky, 1996; Murdaugh, 1981). ("Attenuation" means constriction or reduction.) The correlation between scores on a test and scores on some external gold standard never can be any greater than the square root of the reliability coefficient for the test. In the extreme, if the reliability coefficient is zero, then the validity coefficient also must be zero. Therefore, no reliability implies no criterion-related validity. Note, however, that the converse is not true. Zero validity does not necessarily imply zero reliability. As I pointed out earlier, you could have an instrument that yields very consistent scores but does not properly operationalize any construct.

It should be noted that essay tests and similar "subjective" assessments constitute a counterexample to the claim that a measuring instrument cannot be valid unless it is reliable. Most essay tests often have very strong *content validity* but suffer from poor *interrater reliability* because equally competent judges of essay-writing ability often do not agree regarding the grades that should be assigned.

LEVELS OF MEASUREMENT

About 50 years ago, S. S. Stevens (1946), a Harvard University psychologist, argued that all measurement scales can be subsumed under four types. The first (and most primitive) level he called the **nominal** level. For this type of measurement, all you are able to do is to classify the things being measured into two or more categories. (Variables having just two categories are very common; they are called **dichotomies**.) Numbers may be used as labels for the categories, but such numbers cannot be mathematically manipulated in the same way as can ordinary numbers. They cannot be compared for relative magnitudes; they cannot be added, subtracted, multiplied, or divided; and so on. The simplest example of the nominal level of measurement is sex or gender. The researcher may code male = 1 and female = 2, but any two other numbers would work just as well. (A popular alternative is to use the numbers 0 and 1 to denote the categories of a dichotomy; such a variable is called a **dummy variable**.) A slightly more complicated example would be religious affiliation with, say, Protestant = 1, Catholic = 2, Jewish = 3, and "other" or "none" = 4. Once again, the numbers used have no numerical importance other than to serve as labels for the categories.

The next level Stevens (1946) called **ordinal**. Here the categories are ordered in some meaningful way, and the numbers chosen to represent the various categories also are ordered. For example, it is quite common for hospitals to indicate the conditions of inpatients by using words such as "good," "stable," "guarded," and "critical." Treating this as a measurement problem, you might assign the numbers 1, 2, 3, and 4 to good, stable, guarded, and critical, respectively (or in the reverse order if high scores are "better" than low scores). A patient with a score of 2 on "health condition," "health status," or some such name for the variable not only is of a different condition from a patient with a score of 4 but also is in a more favorable condition. But there is nothing special about the numbers 1, 2, 3, and 4; any four numbers in the same order as 1, 2, 3, and 4 would be equally appropriate as labels for the four health status categories. Like nominal variables, ordinal variables should not be subjected to the usual arithmetical operations, for example, those involved in determining the mean of a set of measurements.

Interval variables constitute the third level. At this level, the categories of the variable are not only different and ordered but also separated by fixed intervals based on an actual unit of measurement. The operationalization of temperature provides the classic example of an interval-level variable. For the Centigrade (Celsius) scale, the categories employed are 0 (the point at which water becomes ice), 1, 2, and so on, but negative values also are possible. For the Fahrenheit scale, the same categories also are used, but the useful range is not the same. (For humans, body temperatures typically range from about 36°C to 40°C and from about 97°F to 104°F.) The zero point on an interval scale always is arbitrary (but not capricious); for example, some event other than water becoming ice could have been chosen as the zero point for Centigrade values. But the important difference between an interval scale and an ordinal scale is the existence of an actual unit of measurement (the *degree* in the case of temperature Centigrade or Fahrenheit) that is constant throughout the entire scale. A difference between 36°C and 37°C is 1°, and that is the same 1° difference as the difference between 37°C and 38°C. Such is not the case for the health status variable treated in the previous paragraph. The difference between a health status rating of 2 and a health status rating of 3 has no meaning whatsoever precisely because such a scale does not even *have* a unit of measurement, much less a unit that is constant throughout the scale.

Because the zero point is arbitrary for an interval scale, it sometimes is convenient to use as a zero point some value other than the one that originally was devised for the scale. For example, you might want to define a variable to be something like the number of degrees above normal body temperature and use numbers such as –1, 0, 1, 2, 3, and 4 rather than 36, 37, 38, 39, 40, and 41 (with a temperature of 37° as the "new" zero point).

The fourth (and most precise) level of measurement is that represented by **ratio** scales that have an absolute rather than arbitrary zero point and for which a score of zero actually means "none" of the quantity being measured. Just as the measurement of body temperature produces the prototypical interval scale, the measurement of body weight produces the prototypical ratio scale. Negative scores are not possible for ratio scales because you cannot have less than nothing of a quantity. Not only are the categories different, ordered, and separated by a constant unit of measurement, but ratio scales also permit interpretations such as that Person A has twice as much of __ (the thing being measured) as does Person B. Such interpretations are unwarranted for interval scales such as temperature (one object is never said to be twice as hot as another) and do not even begin to make sense for ordinal and nominal scales.

One of the simplest, yet often most appropriate, types of ratio scale is a scale that consists of the counting numbers 0, 1, 2, and so on. Sometimes nursing researchers go to great lengths to develop a complicated scale to measure something like smoking behavior, whereas a simple count of number of cigarettes (or number of *packs* of cigarettes) smoked in a given time period (e.g., 1 day) might very well suffice.

So far as levels of measurement are concerned, you always should ask yourself, "What can I say about Mary's score on this measuring instrument?" If all you can say is that her score is different from John's score, then you have nominal measurement. If you also can say that her score is higher than his, then you have ordinal measurement. In addition, if you can say that her score is so many "somethings" higher than his, then the interval level has been attained. Finally, if you also can say that her score is twice or thrice (or whatever) as high as his, then the scale you have employed has met the requirements of a ratio scale.

The most popular type of scale used in nursing research, the ordinal scale, is actually the one that should be avoided whenever possible. Such scales are not very precise and do not lend themselves well to traditional statistical analyses. There is a heated controversy regarding the treatment of ordinal scales as interval scales. I summarized that controversy a few years ago and made an attempt to resolve it (Knapp, 1990, 1993), but the debate continues today.

Table 10.4 Examples of Different Levels of Measurement for the Same
Construct

Level of Measurement	Anatomical Knowledge	Height
Nominal	Identifies bones correctly (1) or incorrectly (2)	64 inches tall (1) or *not* 64 inches tall (2)
Ordinal	Identifies bones very well (1), generally well (2), or poorly (3)	Less than 64 inches tall (1), 64 inches tall (2), or more than 64 inches tall (3)
Interval	Percentage of bones identified correctly that is greater than 60% of possible	Number of inches between top of tennis net and top of head
Ratio	Percentage of bones identified correctly	Number of inches between floor and top of head

I summarize in Table 10.4 how both height and anatomical knowledge could be operationalized at the nominal, ordinal, interval, or ratio level of measurement.

IMPLICATIONS FOR DATA ANALYSIS

It already has been pointed out in the discussion of the ordinal level of measurement that the use of arithmetic means is not appropriate for such scales (see also Marcus-Roberts & Roberts, 1987). The type of scale one happens to have is one of the principal determiners of the types of data analyses that are defensible in research studies in which a given scale is employed. There are certain types of statistical analyses that are perfectly fine for nominal scales, others that require at least ordinal-level scales, still others that can be used with interval or ratio scales, and a few that are reasonable only for ratio scales. This matter is treated in greater detail in Chapter 11, which deals with the statistical analysis of quantitative data.

THE PHYSICAL SCIENCES
COMPARED WITH THE SOCIAL SCIENCES

Validity problems in the physical sciences are very similar to validity problems in the social sciences. Whether or not a thermometer really measures temperature is no easier (and no harder) to determine than is whether or not the McGill Pain Questionnaire really measures pain. But reliability problems are *much* easier in the physical sciences. A thermometer may not measure temperature, but whatever it measures, it does so much more reliably than the McGill Pain Questionnaire measures whatever it measures.

All types of measuring instruments are used in nursing research, ranging from traditional biophysiological equipment such as thermometers and sphygmomanometers to a wide variety of psychosocial devices such as questionnaires and rating scales. I now review some of the "tools" that have been found to be particularly useful in various approaches to theoretical and practical research questions in nursing science.

PHYSICAL SCIENCE INSTRUMENTS

Although I estimate nursing research to be approximately one fourth physical and three fourths social, even the most dyed-in-the-wool social researchers often have need in their studies to measure vital signs, weight, cotinine levels, and so on if for no other reason than to describe the general illness or wellness of the people who are the subjects of their investigations. Perceived degree of comfort, body image, and self-reported smoking behavior all are well and good, but they often require physiological corroboration to properly answer certain interesting research questions such as "What is the relationship between obesity and hypertension?" Studies that combine physical and social approaches to a problem also are highly regarded by funding agencies.

Evaluation of these instruments with respect to validity and reliability requires special care because most of the literature on validity and reliability originated in psychology or education. Consider the matter of an "item," which is so crucial in social measurement. Biophysiological instruments do not have items. When you measure a person's temperature, for example, you get a single number, say 99°F. You do not get item scores that you add together to arrive at a total score on temperature. That just would not make any sense. Because thermometers, yardsticks, and scale balances do not produce item data, all of the techniques for estimating validity and reliability that depend on such data (e.g., factor analyses of interitem correlations, split-half procedures) are not available for judging the goodness or badness of those devices. Of the three principal types of validity considered in the previous chapter, only certain types of content validity and construct validity assessments are appropriate. (There usually is no external gold standard for studying the criterion-related validity of physical measuring instruments.) Because the concept of parallel forms is foreign to physical measurement (Are my electronic thermometer and your electronic thermometer parallel forms?), the only types of reliability that are relevant are test-retest (or measure-remeasure), interrater, and intrarater. But if you think about it, for biophysiological instruments, test-retest, interrater, and intrarater reliability ultimately come down to the same thing. It is just a question of who or what does the measuring the second time.

Interestingly, you hardly ever find physical scientists worrying about validity at all. "Does this thermometer really measure temperature?" rarely is asked. (I think it should be asked.) But they are *very* concerned about the amount of freedom from random measurement error (they usually do not use the term "reliability" either) of their instruments and constantly are calibrating and recalibrating them.

For examples of studies concerned with the validity and reliability of instruments for measuring temperature, see Heidenreich and Giuffre (1990), Heidenreich et al. (1992), and Lattavo, Britt, and Dobal (1995). DeKeyser and Pugh (1990) discussed procedures for investigating the validity and reliability of one type of physical measurement device for measuring biochemical properties, whereas Pugh and DeKeyser (1995) summarized the use of physiological variables in general in nursing research studies published in the period 1989 to 1993. Weiss (1992) discussed similar issues when measuring tactile stimuli. Sommers, Woods, and Courtade (1993) also addressed such issues regarding the assessment of cardiac output. Engstrom (1988) provided a comprehensive treatment of the reliability of physical science instruments in general.

An example of a description of a physical science approach to the measurement of infant pain is found in an article by Franck (1986). She carried out a pilot study to determine whether "photogrammetric" techniques could be used to obtain and evaluate pain responses (to heelstick pricks) by 10 healthy newborns (8 males, 2 females). The device that she employed consisted of several components (table, camera, video recorder, etc.) for recording latency of leg withdrawal, number of leg movements, latency of cry, and other variables assumed to be relevant to infant pain. Such instruments are particularly promising for pain assessment in infants because, unlike adults, they are developmentally incapable of telling us where and how much they hurt.

Another example is provided by Engstrom and Chen's (1984) careful descriptions of a number of extrauterine measurements taken on a sample of 44 women in labor. The purpose of their study was to explore the relationship between certain measures (fundal height, uterine width, abdominal girth, etc.) and infant birthweight. The relationships were then used to derive an equation for predicting birthweights, and those predictions were compared to both the actual birthweights and the predictions obtained from palpation of the maternal abdomen during labor.

A third and very fascinating example is the measurement of voice stress by means of the Psychological Stress Evaluator, a device used by Hurley (1983) to quantify marital conflict. She also used an audio recorder to measure frequency of pauses, frequency of laughter, and other variables for a sample of 68 middle-class married couples. Those variables were hypothesized to be inversely related to marital stress, but the results of the study were actually in the opposite direction. The chapter in Polit and Hungler (1995) that deals with biophysiological methods contains examples of other devices and also addresses ways of determining their measurement properties.

SOCIAL SCIENCE INSTRUMENTS

Because my estimate is that nursing research is approximately 25% physical and 75% social, I devote the rest of this chapter to the types of instruments that are used most frequently in the social side of nursing science. In social research, if you want to measure anything, then you have only three choices: (a) ask, (b) observe, or (c) read records (see Chapter 1). Those are not very technical terms, but because they summarize the situation rather nicely, I use them as the basis for my taxonomy of social measurement.

ASKING

Most social research instruments used in quantitative nursing research are "asking" devices because nursing researchers care about people's perceptions. If we want to find out whether or not patients are in pain or how much pain they are experiencing, then we ask them; if we want to find out the sizes of their social support networks, then we ask them; and so on. But the particular form that the asking device takes varies considerably. Some researchers use only carefully standardized tests for which there are established norms and extensive validity and reliability data (e.g., the NLN Achievement Test). Others prefer unstructured and unstandardized interviews (similar to typical clinical interviews). There are a number of intermediate positions as well.

Asking instruments usually consist of several items for which individual item scores are obtained, with those scores subsequently summed or averaged to produce subscale scores and/or total scores. But there are many examples of instruments that consist of just one item. (See Youngblot & Casper, 1993, for a defense of single-item indicators.)

One single-item instrument that is similar to a standardized test is the **visual analogue scale.** When this type of scale is used, the respondent is asked to indicate by putting a mark on a scale ranging from 0 to 100 his or her position, attitude, feelings, and so on with respect to a particular matter that is of interest to the researcher. A visual analogue scale is "standardized" in the sense that it almost always is 10 centimeters in length and the directions for using it are essentially constant from one study to another, but there are no norms. For a thorough discussion of visual analogue scales including some of their advantages and disadvantages, see Cline, Herman, Shaw, and Morton (1992); Lee and Kieckhefer (1989); and Wewers and Lowe (1990). For a recent example of a study that was concerned with the selection of a "best" visual analogue scale for measuring children's and adolescents' pain intensity, see Tesler et al. (1991). For an interesting example of the actual use of visual analogue scales, see Simpson, Lee, and Cameron (1996).

An instrument that is somewhat further removed from a standardized test is the **semantic differential** developed by Osgood, Suci, and Tannenbaum (1957). The technique is standardized only in the sense that people always are given a number of concepts such as nurse, caring, and death and are asked to rate each of them on a set of bipolar adjectival scales such as good-bad or strong-weak, but the concepts and scales differ from study to study and there are no norms. (For examples of applications of the semantic differential methodology to nursing research, see the later discussion in this chapter of the studies carried out by Morgan, 1984, and Bowles, 1986.)

Semantic differential scales are variations on scales originally suggested by Rensis Likert (1932). The principal difference between **Likert-type scales** and semantic differential scales is that the former typically have five ordinal response options with *strongly agree* and *strongly disagree* as the endpoints and *agree, undecided,* and *disagree* as the intermediate points, whereas the latter typically have seven options with an adjective (e.g., *good*) at one end and its antonym (e.g., *bad*) at the other end and five other spaces in between without labels but representing varying degrees of intensity. For an interesting example of a Likert-type scale, see Froman and Owen (1997). For a critique of the use of Likert-type scales with people of various cultures, see Flaskerud (1988).

The researcher always should make it perfectly clear who the "ask*er*" and "ask*ee*" are. This is particularly true when the focus is on *perceptions*. When attempting to measure pediatric pain, for example, the consumer of the research findings needs to know who was asking whose perception of whose pain because different persons' perceptions of the same phenomenon do not always agree. The asker usually is the attending nurse or nurse researcher but could very well be the parent. The askee ideally should be the child, of course, but because very young children are unable to respond verbally, the nurse researcher might ask the child's mother what her perception is of the amount or type of pain that she thinks the child is experiencing. As an example of the asker/askee specification for a non-pain situation, Koniak-Griffin and Ludington-Hoe (1988) asked a sample of 81 mothers to rate their infants' temperament at 4 months and 8 months of age on each of ninety-five 6-point Likert-type scales.

Far and away, the most common form of asking used in nursing research is the printed questionnaire. Sometimes questionnaires are administered "live" to a group of subjects assembled for that purpose. More often, they are mailed out by the researcher, filled out (or, alas, ignored or thrown away!) by the respondents, and mailed back. Questionnaires may seem to be an easy way in which to get data, but they are actually very difficult to construct and suffer from all types of problems, not the least of which is the problem of nonresponse. For other strengths and weaknesses of questionnaires, particularly those that involve using the mail service, see Topf (1986a) and Woolley (1984).

An interview schedule is similar to a questionnaire, but the measurement setting is a one-on-one situation in which the interviewer poses a set of questions to a respondent and the respondent is able to clarify, and expand on, the answers given. In an unstructured interview, however, the questions are not predetermined or constant for all subjects. Investigators who favor the unstructured interview argue that asking the same questions of all respondents constrains the research unnecessarily and may miss certain valuable bits of information.

One of the simplest interview schedules ever used in nursing research is the list of medical terms compiled by Byrne and Edeani (1984). They individually interviewed 125 patients in a county general hospital and gave each of them a multiple-choice test consisting of 50 randomly selected terms followed by three answers, one of which was correct (source: *Taber's Cyclopedic Medical Dictionary*) and two of which were incorrect. The percentage correct ranged from 10.4% (for "mastectomy") to 96.0% (for "autopsy"). A few years later, Spees (1991) tested the knowledge of the same terms when she interviewed 25 clients and 25 family members. The percentage correct for her sample ranged from 68.0% (for "emesis") to 100.0% (for "abnormal," "complication," "diagnosis," "gastric ulcer," "hypertension," "injection," "intravenous," "nausea," and "surgeon"). These are just two examples of a fairly large literature on what might be called "health care literacy." Some researchers incorrectly assume that subjects in their investigations are familiar with terms that often are unknown to the average person.

RATING VERSUS RANKING

A very common confusion in the research literature is the matter of rating versus ranking. I already have referred to ratings at some length. Ratings are the categories of ordinal scales. You might ask a physician to rate the condition of each of 10 patients on a 4-point scale such as 1 = *good,* 2 = *stable,* 3 = *guarded,* and 4 = *critical.* Any combination of 1's, 2's, 3's, and 4's might result.

Rankings are a different matter entirely. They are measurements that always go from 1 to *N,* where *N* is the number of things being ranked. If you asked that same physician to *rank* the 10 patients' conditions, the patient in the best condition would get Rank 1, the patient in the next best condition would get Rank 2, and so on down to the patient in the worst condition who would get Rank 10, no matter how sick or well in some absolute sense the patients may happen to be.

"ASKING" EXAMPLES

Two very interesting but very different ways of measuring by asking are the semantic differential technique and Q sorts, originating with Stephenson (1953) and summarized nicely by Dennis (1986, 1987, 1988, 1990). I now describe two studies that used the semantic differential approach and two that used Q sorts. Although neither procedure has been used very frequently in nursing research to date (Strickland & Waltz, 1986, counted only three instances of the semantic differential and one Q sort out of 385 measuring formats reported in 99 articles appearing in 1984 in *Nursing Research, International Journal of Nursing Studies,* and *Research in Nursing & Health*), both hold great promise for future use.

Attitudes of white nursing students toward black patients were of interest to Morgan (1984). She asked a sample of 242 senior nursing students to rate each of the concepts "ideal person," "black American," "black American patient," "white American," and "white American patient" on each of 20 bipolar adjectival scales. Of the 20 scales, 10 (e.g., good-bad) represented Osgood et al.'s "evaluation" factor, 5 (e.g., strong-weak) represented the "potency" factor, and 5 (e.g., fast-slow) represented the "activity" factor. Morgan investigated the significance of the differences between various pairs of concepts and determined that the only *nonsignificant* difference was between white American and white American patient. Of particular concern was the finding that nursing students perceived white American patient more positively than black American patient.

Bowles (1986) wanted to measure women's attitudes toward menopause. She also chose the semantic differential approach. For her instrument, Bowles used only the single concept "menopause" (understandably enough) and an initial set of 45 scales thought to be relevant to the assessment of the attitudes in which she was interested. Some were selected from the original work of Osgood et al. (1957), others were drawn from the general literature on menopause, and still others were taken directly from two other studies of menopause that also used the semantic differential. On the basis of two factor analyses of the responses of 504 adult females in northern Illinois, the 45 scales were reduced to 20 scales, all of which were indicators of the "evaluative" dimension underlying attitudes toward menopause. Although the main purpose of her study was methodological (to develop and validate her instrument), she did find that subjects

35 years of age or younger expressed more negative feelings toward menopause than did subjects older than 35 years of age.

Following on her summary of Q methodology in *Advances in Nursing Science* in 1986, Dennis (1987) reported the results of a substantive study that used Q sorts in an article published in *Nursing Research*. In the study, 60 medical-surgical patients were asked to sort 45 "client control" items (e.g., "contribute to discussions about whether or not to have certain diagnostic tests") into 11 categories with a predetermined number of items to be placed in each category; that is, each patient was "forced" to put a certain number of items in each of the categories but was "free" to choose *which* items to place in which categories. The patients performed the Q sort twice, once with respect to what was important to them regarding getting well and going home and then with respect to what was important to them regarding making their hospital stays more pleasant. The following year, Dennis (1988) contributed a chapter on Q methodology in the second volume of Strickland and Waltz's work on the measurement of nursing outcomes. Two years later, she reported the results of another study that also used Q methodology (Dennis, 1990).

Q technique also was used by Stokes and Gordon (1988) to measure stress in the elderly. Each askee (in this case, members of two small convenience samples in Florida and New York) sorted 104 stressors into nine categories with verbal labels ranging from *least stressful* to *most stressful*. Like Bowles (1986), their contribution was primarily methodological (the psychometric evaluation of an instrument called the Stokes-Gordon Stress Scale [SGSS]), but they obtained some interesting substantive results. They found that scores on the SGSS correlated positively and significantly with onset of illnesses for the total year. Stokes and Gordon (1988) called that finding evidence of predictive validity, but it is nothing of the kind given that onset of illness is not a gold standard against which a measure of stress can be validated.

For more on Q sorts, see McKeown and Thomas (1988) and Simpson (1989). For another interesting study of an asking instrument, the Work Assessment Scale, see Gulick (1991).

OBSERVING

The pediatric pain example suggests that asking may not be an appropriate measurement strategy for infant subjects (and for many others, such as Alzheimer's disease patients, where the mere process of asking might change the phenomenon that is being studied). Researchers often choose to actually observe the behavior in which they are interested rather than ask about it. Some research methodologists argue that there is far too much obtrusive asking in social research and not nearly enough unobtrusive observing. (For some very creative approaches to certain research questions for which most researchers would automatically default to traditional questionnaires or interviews but which can be equally well addressed by observation, see Webb, Campbell, Schwartz, Sechrest, & Grove, 1981.) Better yet is a "triangulation" approach (Hinds & Young, 1987; Kimchi, Polivka, & Stevenson, 1991; Mitchell, 1986) that involves both asking *and* observing. If asking about a particular phenomenon and observing it produce comparable results, then the existence of the phenomenon is more firmly established. If the two do not agree, however, then you have a serious validity problem. For example, if a questionnaire or interview approach suggests that there is very little racial prejudice in a community but observation suggests that there is a great deal of racial prejudice in that community, then the researcher must decide which of the two is the more valid measure—a person's perception of his or her behavior or the observed behavior of that person.

Participant observation is a favorite technique of some social scientists. But much observational research in nursing entails a nonparticipant role on the part of the investigator. A good example of the latter is to be found in much of maternal-child research, which often uses "one-way mirror" observation of interactions between mother and infant.

Instruments for recording observational data, like asking instruments, range from highly structured standardized devices such as the Brazelton Neonatal Behavioral Assessment Scale to unstructured researcher-constructed field note ledgers and checklists with something like the Apgar as an intermediate example. Issues of interrater reliability are especially crucial for observational measurement ("Do you see what I see?").

"OBSERVING" EXAMPLES

Reference already has been made to the study of infant temperament by Koniak-Griffin and Ludington-Hoe (1988). In addition to asking the mothers to rate their infants' temperament, the investigators used the standardized Bayley Scales of Infant Development to observe and record psychomotor development at both 4 months and 8 months of age.

Earlier work by Schraeder and Medoff-Cooper (1983) that also was concerned with infant development and temperament made use of the Denver Developmental Screening Test to measure gross and fine motor abilities and the Home Observation for Measurement of the Environment to measure various aspects of the child-rearing environment. The primary purpose of their research was the determination of the "at-risk" (for developmental delay) percentage of a small sample of 26 children who had been followed up in a 2-year longitudinal study.

A third example of measurement by observation, and again for infants, is the study by Medoff-Cooper and Brooten (1987) of a very small sample of nine premature babies. The authors were interested in how different points in the feeding cycle related to neurobehavioral assessment. They observed the infants on a variety of dimensions including level of consciousness, posture, and irritability on each of three occasions (1 hour before feeding, 10 minutes before the next feeding, and 1 hour before the third feeding). They found few relationships between time and neurobehavior, with most of the assessments quite stable across the various occasions.

A final example is the work by Larson et al. (1996) of the psychometric characteristics of an instrument designed for use by nurses in assessing the functional status of patients with chronic obstructive pulmonary disease.

READING RECORDS

Certain social researchers (e.g., economists) hardly ever either ask or observe. They "tap into" data that are collected by other researchers (occasionally) or by government officials (more commonly) who have either asked or observed to get the information in the first place. Economists, demographers, historians, and political scientists are frequent "dredgers" of census reports, vital statistics files, voter registration records, and other "data banks." Such sources often contain more valid and reliable information than can be obtained by primary researchers. But sometimes they do not; it is at least awkward to have to rely on other people's definitions and operationalizations. A case in point is inpatients' medical charts. It is very easy, and frequently sufficient, to look up certain information on the charts (e.g., numbers and types of medications) rather than asking patients about such matters or spending hours observing them taking their various medications. But if the researcher is actually interested in *compliance* (Did the patients actually take the medications or did they throw them in the wastebasket?), then the desired information may not appear in the charts.

"READING RECORDS" EXAMPLES

Reading records is a strategy often used in secondary analyses of research data (see Chapter 13). To test a particular model of health behavior, Cox, Sullivan, and Roghmann (1984) used a data bank previously collected by survey researchers concerned with prenatal screening. In their research, Cox et al. extracted from that existing file measures of a number of characteristics of 203 women (e.g., age, education, type of insurance coverage) that were hypothesized to influence their acceptance or rejection of amniocentesis (the dependent variable). They also constructed a few other measures (e.g., attitude toward legalized abortion) by creating an index based on some item data that were part of the file.

A study by Powers and Jalowiec (1987) used a chart review to obtain dietary information and health histories for a sample of 450 hypertensive patients randomly selected from the Chicago area. They also interviewed those same patients to get some additional information about diet and health histories and for measuring other variables in which they were interested such as locus of control and quality of life.

An unusual article that addressed the validity and reliability of one reading records measurement source, health diaries, is that by Burman (1995). Individual record keepers *provide* the data; researchers look up the data in the records. For more on the reliability of health diaries, see Rogers, Caruso, and Aldrich (1993). For a general article regarding the use of health diaries with children, see Butz and Alexander (1991).

AN INTERESTING "COMBINATION" PHYSICAL-SOCIAL EXAMPLE

Voda, Inle, and Atwood (1980) adopted a physical science approach to the quantification of a social science measurement problem: self-report of the location of menopausal hot flash. Each member of a sample of menopausal women was given a piece of 8½ × 11-inch paper depicting two pairs of body diagrams of a female figure, with each pair consisting of a front view and a back view, and was asked to shade in on one pair of front and back diagrams the part(s) of her body where the hot flash originated and to shade in on the other pair of diagrams the part(s) of her body to which the hot flash had spread. To quantify the amount of flash, the authors used two different techniques. The first involved cutting out the shaded areas, weighing them (on a sensitive balance scale), and determining the proportion of the full figure weight (which had been determined previously) for both the origin and the spread of the flash. The second technique involved tracing around the edges of the shaded areas with a compensating polar planimeter and determining the proportion of the full figure area (again, as determined previously) constituted by the origin and the spread. The authors included a fascinating discussion of procedures for determining the validity and reliability of these measuring instruments, and they suggested some applications other than the assessment of self-reported hot flashes. One cannot help but be impressed by the care that went into this unusual form of nursing instrumentation.

SOME FINAL NOTES
REGARDING MEASUREMENT

It is quite common to find tests of significance carried out on validity and reliability coefficients. That is fine so long as it is clearly understood that statistical significance may be necessary but is far from sufficient. For example, a test-retest reliability coefficient of .18, based on a sample size of 200 subjects, is statistically significant at the .05 level but is indicative of very poor instrument stability.

A common error in research is the confusion of a variable with a category of a variable. For example, self-reported sex is a variable; female is a category of that variable. When making statements about the relationship between any two things, you always should phrase the statement in terms of variables rather than their categories. It is correct to say that there is a relationship between religious affiliation and political affiliation (assuming that there is); it is incorrect to say that there is a relationship between being Catholic and being a Democrat (even if all Catholics are Democrats or if all Democrats are Catholics). You can have an *association* between a category of one variable and a category of another variable, but a relationship always holds between one variable and another variable.

You will find in the nursing research literature several references to "rules" regarding minimum values for reliability coefficients, minimum numbers of observations per variable, and the like. Most of such rules are quite arbitrary and should be "taken with a grain of salt" (see Knapp & Brown, 1995).

Although I believe that this discussion has covered the principal types of measuring instruments used in nursing research, I have by no stretch of the imagination exhausted all of the variations on the basic types. The pages of *Nursing Research* and other scholarly journals reflect a wide range of instruments that have been or could be used to operationalize all sorts of interesting nursing constructs. If you find yourself embarking on a research project and you think you may have to make up your own measuring instrument, then think again. Chances are that someone else already has beaten you to it and can save you a lot of work.

Think of measurement as a gigantic leap between truth and its manifestation. "God knows" not only what the true reading is on the particular thermometer that you happen to have in your mouth but also what your body temperature really is. We mere mortals can at best only approximate both.

REFERENCES

Abraham, I. L. (1994). Does suboptimal measurement reliability constrain the explained variance in regression? *Western Journal of Nursing Research, 16,* 447-452.

Armstrong, G. D. (1981). The intraclass correlation as a measure of interrater reliability of subjective judgments. *Nursing Research, 30,* 314-320.

Berk, R. A. (1990). Importance of expert judgment in content-related validity evidence. *Western Journal of Nursing Research, 12,* 659-671.

Beyer, J. E., & Aradine, C. R. (1986). Content validity of an instrument to measure young children's perceptions of the intensity of their pain. *Journal of Pediatric Nursing, 1,* 386-395.

Beyer, J. E., & Aradine, C. R. (1988). Convergent and discriminant validity of a self-report measure of pain intensity for children. *Children's Health Care, 16,* 274-282.

Beyer, J. E., & Knapp, T. R. (1986). Methodological issues in the measurement of children's pain. *Children's Health Care, 14,* 233-241.

Bowles, C. (1986). Measure of attitude toward menopause using the semantic differential model. *Nursing Research, 35,* 81-86.

Burman, M. E. (1995). Health diaries in nursing research and practice. *Image, 27,* 147-152.

Butz, A. M., & Alexander, C. (1991). Use of health diaries with children. *Nursing Research, 40,* 59-61.

Byra-Cook, C. J., Dracup, K. A., & Lazik, A. J. (1990). Direct and indirect blood pressure in critical care patients. *Nursing Research, 39,* 285-288.

Byrne, T. J., & Edeani, D. (1984). Knowledge of medical terminology among hospital patients. *Nursing Research, 33,* 178-181.

Campbell, D. T., & Fiske, D. W. (1959). Convergent and discriminant validation by the multitrait-multimethod matrix. *Psychological Bulletin, 56,* 81-105.

Cline, M. E., Herman, J., Shaw, E. R., & Morton, R. D. (1992). Standardization of the visual analogue scale. *Nursing Research, 41,* 378-380.

Cohen, J. (1960). A coefficient of agreement for nominal scales. *Educational and Psychological Measurement, 20,* 37-46.

Cox, C. L., Sullivan, J. A., & Roghmann, K. J. (1984). A conceptual explanation of risk-reduction behavior and intervention development. *Nursing Research, 33,* 168-173.

Cronbach, L. J. (1951). Coefficient alpha and the internal structure of tests. *Psychometrika, 16,* 297-334.

DeKeyser, F. G., & Pugh, L. C. (1990). Assessment of the reliability and validity of biochemical measures. *Nursing Research, 39,* 314-316.

Dennis, K. E. (1986). Q methodology: Relevance and application to nursing research. *Advances in Nursing Science, 8*(3), 6-17.

Dennis, K. E. (1987). Dimensions of client control. *Nursing Research, 36,* 151-156.

Dennis, K. E. (1988). Q methodology: New perspectives on estimating reliability and validity. In O. L. Strickland & C. F. Waltz (Eds.), *Measurement of nursing outcomes,* Vol. 2: *Measuring nursing performance* (pp. 409-419). New York: Springer.

Dennis, K. E. (1990). Patients' control and the information imperative: Clarification and confirmation. *Nursing Research, 39,* 162-166.

England, M., & Roberts, B. L. (1996). Theoretical and psychometric analysis of caregiver strain. *Research in Nursing & Health, 19,* 499-510.

Engstrom, J. L. (1988). Assessment of the reliability of physical measures. *Research in Nursing & Health, 11,* 383-389.

Engstrom, J. L., & Chen, E. H. (1984). Prediction of birthweight by the use of extrauterine measurements during labor. *Research in Nursing & Health, 7,* 314-323.

Fawcett, J., & Knauth, D. (1996). The factor structure of the Perception of Birth Scale. *Nursing Research, 45,* 83-86.

Flaskerud, J. H. (1988). Is the Likert scale format culturally biased? *Nursing Research, 37,* 185-186.

Fox, R. N. (1982). Agreement corrected for chance. *Research in Nursing & Health, 5,* 45-46.

Franck, L. S. (1986). A new method to quantitatively describe pain behavior in infants. *Nursing Research, 35,* 28-31.

Froman, R. D., & Owen, S. V. (1997). Further validation of the AIDS Attitude Scale. *Research in Nursing & Health, 20,* 161-167.

Goldsmith, J. W. (1981). Methodological considerations in using videotape to establish rater reliability. *Nursing Research, 30,* 124-127.

Goodwin, L. D., & Prescott, P. A. (1981). Issues and approaches to estimating interrater reliability in nursing research. *Research in Nursing & Health, 4,* 323-337.

Gross, D. (1991). Issues related to validity of videotaped observational data. *Western Journal of Nursing Research, 13,* 658-663.

Gross, D., Conrad, B., Fogg, L., Willis, L., & Garvey, C. (1993). What does the NCATS measure? *Nursing Research, 42,* 260-265.

Gulick, E. E. (1991). Reliability and validity of the Work Assessment Scale for persons with multiple sclerosis. *Nursing Research, 40,* 107-112.

Guttman, L. (1941). The quantification of a class of attributes: A theory and method for scale construction. In P. Horst (Ed.), *The prediction of personal adjustment* (pp. 319-348). New York: Social Science Research Council.

Heidenreich, T., & Giuffre, M. (1990). Postoperative temperature measurement. *Nursing Research, 39,* 153-155.

Heidenreich, T., Giuffre, M., & Doorley, J. (1992). Temperature and temperature measurement after induced hypothermia. *Nursing Research, 41,* 296-300.

Heise, D. R. (1969). Separating reliability and stability in test-retest correlation. *American Sociological Review, 34,* 93-101.

Hinds, P. S., & Young, K. J. (1987). A triangulation of methods and paradigms to study nurse-given wellness care. *Nursing Research, 36,* 195-198.

Hurley, P. M. (1983). Communication variables and voice analysis of marital conflict stress. *Nursing Research, 32,* 164-169.

Jacobsen, B. S., Tulman, L., & Lowery, B. J. (1991). Three sides of the same coin: The analysis of paired data from dyads. *Nursing Research, 40,* 359-363.

Jones, E. (1987). Translation of quantitative measures for use in cross-cultural research. *Nursing Research, 36,* 324-327.

Kimchi, J., Polivka, B., & Stevenson, J. S. (1991). Triangulation: Operational definitions. *Nursing Research, 40,* 364-366.

Knapp, T. R. (1985). Validity, reliability, and neither. *Nursing Research, 37,* 189-192.

Knapp, T. R. (1988). Stress versus strain: A methodological critique. *Nursing Research, 37,* 181-184.

Knapp, T. R. (1990). Treating ordinal scales as interval scales: An attempt to resolve the controversy. *Nursing Research, 39,* 121-123.

Knapp, T. R. (1991). Coefficient alpha: Conceptualizations and anomalies. *Research in Nursing & Health, 14,* 457-460.

Knapp, T. R. (1993). Treating ordinal scales as ordinal scales. *Nursing Research, 42,* 184-186.

Knapp, T. R., & Brown, J. K. (1995). Ten measurement commandments that often should be broken. *Research in Nursing & Health, 18,* 465-469.

Knapp, T. R., Kimble, L. P., & Dunbar, S. B. (1998). Distinguishing between the stability of a construct and the stability of an instrument in trait/state measurement. *Nursing Research.*

Koniak-Griffin, S., & Ludington-Hoe, S. M. (1988). Developmental and temperament outcomes of sensory stimulation in healthy infants. *Nursing Research, 37,* 70-76.

Larson, E. (1986). Evaluating validity of screening tests. *Nursing Research, 35,* 186-188.

Larson, J. L., Covey, M. K., Vitalo, C. A., Alex, C. G., Patel, M., & Kim, M. J. (1996). Reliability and validity of the 12-minute distance walk in patients with chronic obstructive pulmonary disease. *Nursing Research, 45,* 203-210.

Lattavo, K., Britt, J., & Dobal, M. (1995). Agreement between measures of pulmonary artery and tympanic temperatures. *Research in Nursing & Health, 18,* 365-370.

Lee, K. A., & Kieckhefer, G. M. (1989). Measuring human responses using visual analogue scales. *Western Journal of Nursing Research, 11,* 128-132.

Leidy, N. K., Abbott, R. D., & Fedenko, K. M. (1997). Sensitivity and reproducibility of the dual-mode actigraph under controlled levels of activity intensity. *Nursing Research, 46,* 5-11.

Likert, R. (1932). A technique for the assessment of attitudes. *Archives of Psychology, 22,* 5-55.

Lowe, N. K., Walker, S. N., & MacCallum, R. C. (1991). Confirming the theoretical structure of the McGill Pain Questionnaire in acute clinical pain. *Pain, 46,* 53-60.

Lynn, M. R. (1986). Determination and quantification of content validity. *Nursing Research, 35,* 382-385.

Mahon, N. E., Yarcheski, T. J., & Yarcheski, A. (1995). Validation of the Revised UCLA Loneliness Scale for adolescents. *Research in Nursing & Health, 18,* 263-270.

Marcus-Roberts, H., & Roberts, F. (1987). Meaningless statistics. *Journal of Educational Statistics, 12,* 383-394.

McGuire, D. (1984). The measurement of clinical pain. *Nursing Research, 33,* 152-156.

McKeown, B., & Thomas, D. (1988). *Q methodology.* Newbury Park, CA: Sage.

Medoff-Cooper, B., & Brooten, D. (1987). Relation of the feeding cycle to neurobehavioral assessment in preterm infants: A pilot study. *Nursing Research, 36,* 315-317.

Mitchell, E. S. (1986). Multiple triangulation: A methodology for nursing science. *Advances in Nursing Science, 8*(3), 18-26.

Morgan, B. S. (1984). A semantic differential measure of attitudes toward black American patients. *Research in Nursing & Health, 7,* 155-162.

Muchinsky, P. M. (1996). The correction for attenuation. *Educational and Psychological Measurement, 56,* 63-75.

Munro, B. H. (1997). *Statistics for health care research* (3rd ed.). Philadelphia: Lippincott.

Murdaugh, C. (1981). Measurement error and attenuation. *Western Journal of Nursing Research, 3,* 252-256.

Nevo, B. (1985). Face validity revisited. *Journal of Educational Measurement, 22,* 287-293.

Nield, M., & Gocka, I. (1993). To correlate or not to correlate: What is the question? *Nursing Research, 42,* 294-296.

Norbeck, J. S., Lindsey, A. M., & Carrieri, V. L. (1981). The development of an instrument to measure social support. *Nursing Research, 30,* 264-269.

Norbeck, J. S., Lindsey, A. M., & Carrieri, V. L. (1983). Further development of the Norbeck Social Support Questionnaire: Normative data and validity testing. *Nursing Research, 32,* 4-9.

Nunnally, J. C., & Bernstein, I. H. (1994). *Psychometric theory* (3rd ed.). New York: McGraw-Hill.

Osgood, C., Suci, G., & Tannenbaum, P. (1957). *The measurement of meaning.* Urbana: University of Illinois Press.

Padilla, G. V. (1984). Reliability and validity of the independent variable. *Western Journal of Nursing Research, 6,* 138-140.

Polit, D. F., & Hungler, B. P. (1995). *Nursing research: Principles and methods* (5th ed.). Philadelphia: Lippincott.

Powers, M. J., & Jalowiec, A. (1987). Profile of the well-controlled, well-adjusted hypertensive patient. *Nursing Research, 36,* 106-110.

Pugh, L. C., & DeKeyser, F. G. (1995). Use of physiologic variables in nursing research. *Image, 27,* 273-276.

Puntillo, K., & Weiss, S. J. (1994). Pain: Its mediators and associated morbidity in critically ill cardiovascular surgical patients. *Nursing Research, 43,* 31-36.

Rock, D. L., Green, K. E., Wise, B. K., & Rock, R. D. (1984). Social support and social network scales: A psychometric review. *Research in Nursing & Health, 7,* 325-332.

Rogers, A. E., Caruso, C. C., & Aldrich, M. (1993). Reliability of sleep diaries for assessment of sleep/wake patterns. *Nursing Research, 42,* 368-371.

Ryan-Wenger, N. M. (1990). Development and psychometric properties of the Schoolagers' Coping Strategies Inventory. *Nursing Research, 39,* 344-349.

Schraeder, B. D., & Medoff-Cooper, B. (1983). Development and temperament in very low birth weight infants: The second year. *Nursing Research, 32,* 331-335.

Sccolsky, C. (1987). On the direct measurement of face validity: A comment on Nevo. *Journal of Educational Measurement, 24,* 82-83.

Shacham, S., & Daut, R. (1981). Anxiety or pain: What does the scale measure? *Journal of Consulting and Clinical Psychology, 49,* 468-469.

Simpson, S. H. (1989). Use of Q-sort methodology in cross-cultural nutrition and health research. *Nursing Research, 38,* 289-290.

Simpson, T., Lee, E. R., & Cameron, C. (1996). Relationships among sleep dimensions and factors that impair sleep after cardiac surgery. *Research in Nursing & Health, 19,* 213-223.

Sommers, M. S., Woods, S. L., & Courtade, M. A. (1993). Issues in methods and measurement of thermodilution cardiac output. *Nursing Research, 42,* 228-233.

Spees, C. M. (1991). Knowledge of medical terminology among clients and families. *Image, 23,* 225-229.

Spence Laschinger, H. K. (1992). Intraclass correlations as estimates of interrater reliability in nursing research. *Western Journal of Nursing Research, 14,* 246-251.

Stephenson, W. (1953). *The study of behavior: Q-technique and its methodology.* Chicago: University of Chicago Press.

Stevens, S. S. (1946). On the theory of scales of measurement. *Science, 103,* 677-680.

Stokes, S. A., & Gordon, S. E. (1988). Development of an instrument to measure stress in the older adult. *Nursing Research, 37,* 16-19.

Strickland, O. L., & Waltz, C. F. (1986). Measurement of research variables in nursing. In P. L. Chinn (Ed.), *Nursing research methodology* (pp. 79-90). Rockville, MD: Aspen.

Tesler, M. D., Savedra, M. C., Holzemer, W. L., Wilkie, D. J., Ward, J. A., & Paul, S. M. (1991). The word-graphic rating scale as a measure of children's and adolescents' pain intensity. *Research in Nursing & Health, 14,* 361-371.

Thomas, S. D., Hathaway, D. K., & Arheart, K. L. (1992). Face validity. *Western Journal of Nursing Research, 14,* 109-112.

Tilden, V. P., Nelson, C. A., & May, B. A. (1990). Use of qualitative methods to enhance content validity. *Nursing Research, 39,* 172-175.

Topf, M. (1986a). Response sets in questionnaire research. *Nursing Research, 35,* 119-121.

Topf, M. (1986b). Three estimates of interrater reliability for nominal data. *Nursing Research, 35,* 253-255.

Ventura, M. R., Hageman, P. T., Slakter, M. J., & Fox, R. N. (1980). Interrater reliabilities for two measures of nursing care quality. *Research in Nursing & Health, 3,* 25-32.

Voda, A. M., Inle, M., & Atwood, J. R. (1980). Quantification of self-report data from two-dimensional body diagrams. *Western Journal of Nursing Research, 2,* 707-729.

Walker, S. N., Kerr, M. J., Pender, N. J., & Sechrist, K. R. (1990). A Spanish language version of the Health-Promoting Lifestyle Profile. *Nursing Research, 39,* 268-273.

Waltz, C. F., Strickland, O. L., & Lenz, E. R. (1991). *Measurement in nursing research* (2nd ed.). Philadelphia: Davis.

Webb, E. J., Campbell, D. T., Schwartz, R. B., Sechrest, L., & Grove, J. B. (1981). *Nonreactive measures in the social sciences* (2nd ed.). Boston: Houghton Mifflin.

Weinert, C., & Tilden, V. P. (1990). Measures of social support. *Nursing Research, 39,* 212-216.

Weiss, S. J. (1992). Measurement of the sensory qualities in tactile interaction. *Nursing Research, 41,* 82-86.

Wewers, M. E., & Lowe, N. K. (1990). A critical review of visual analogue scales in the measurement of clinical phenomena. *Research in Nursing & Health, 13,* 227-236.

Wineman, N. M., Durand, E. J., & McCulloch, B. J. (1994). Examination of the factor structure of the Ways of Coping Questionnaire with clinical populations. *Nursing Research, 43,* 268-273.

Woolley, A. S. (1984). Questioning the mailed questionnaire as a valid instrument for research in nursing education. *Image, 16,* 115-119.

Youngblot, J. M., & Casper, G. R. (1993). Single-item indicators in nursing research. *Research in Nursing & Health, 16,* 459-465.

STUDY SUGGESTIONS

1. For the article you chose for the study suggestion at the end of Chapter 9, select one of the dimensions (preferably the characteristic of principal interest to the researcher[s]) and identify what the construct is and how it was operationalized (the variable). Do you think that variable was a good operationalization of the construct? Why or why not?

2. Do the obtained scores on that variable constitute a nominal, ordinal, interval, or ratio scale? Why?

3. What evidence is provided for the validity of the instrument that produced the data for that variable? For its reliability? Is such evidence appropriate? Is it sufficient? Why or why not?

4. In your area of specialization or research interest, is physical measurement or social measurement more appropriate? If physical, what instruments are of particular concern to you and what are their strengths and weaknesses? If social, is asking, observing, or reading records the dominant strategy? Why?

5. Read one article that reported the use of the semantic differential and one article that reported the use of Q sorts (not the articles that have been cited in this chapter). Choose the study that you think used the more appropriate approach and explain why.

Statistics

Key Terms: descriptive statistics, inferential statistics, frequency distribution, cross-tabulation (contingency table), contingency coefficient, scatter plot (scatter diagram), Pearson product-moment correlation coefficient, parameter, statistic, interval estimation, hypothesis testing, parametric test, nonparametric test, chi-square test, *t* test, null hypothesis, statistically significant result, regression analysis, regression equation, multiple regression analysis, slope, intercept, multiple correlation coefficient, simultaneous regression, hierarchical regression, covariate, stepwise regression, logistic regression, path model, path coefficient, direct "effect," indirect "effect," path analysis, structural equation modeling

One of the most dreaded aspects of quantitative nursing research is statistics—both using them and reading about them. That is unfortunate because the basic concepts in statistics are rather simple. It is doubly unfortunate because the statistical part of research also is one of the least important parts. A well-designed study that uses good measuring instruments does not need much in the way of statistics to properly interpret the results, and fancy statistical analysis never can salvage a poorly designed study based on bad instruments.

THE ROLE OF STATISTICS
IN NURSING RESEARCH

There are two points in the research process where statistical considerations arise. The first is in conjunction with the design of the study, where issues of sampling, instrument validity and reliability, and a few other methodological matters need to be addressed. Most of these matters already have been treated in this book. In the sampling chapter (Chapter 9), I discussed the notion of a probability sample in general and a simple random sample in particular. I also talked about sample size, a crucial issue when it comes to generalizing from sample to population. Validity and reliability received special emphasis in Chapter 10. As I pointed out in that chapter, reliability is almost totally a statistical phenomenon. Other statistically based principles such as random assignment to treatment groups were subsumed under more general topics in Chapters 3 and 5.

The second and more visible point is in the treatment of the data that are actually obtained in the study proper. It is to this second use that the remainder of this chapter is devoted. But first, I include a brief diversion.

PERCENTAGES

Everybody knows what percentages are. I have talked a little bit about them already (e.g., see Chapter 6), and I have much more to say about them in this chapter because percentages are very important statistics. But they can be tricky, so a few cautions are in order.

First, they always must add to 100. That may sound like a most obvious and trivial concern, but it is surprising how often they do not. One reason is rounding error. It can be remedied by carrying out the calculations to a larger number of decimal places, but this can be annoying. (Is 20 out of 30 equal to 66%, 67%, 66.6%, 66.7%, 66.66%, or 66.67%?) Another reason has to do with nonindependent observations that arise in certain situations such as overlapping groups of patients suffering from various ailments. Percentage lung cancer plus percentage AIDS plus percentage hypertension might very well add to more than 100 if some patients have been diagnosed as having two or more of those problems. A third reason concerns missing data. If religious preference is being analyzed, then there could be some subjects for whom such information is unavailable, and the percentages for the various religions will add to some number less than 100 even if the categories "other" and "none" are included. They could be be made to add to 100 if the number of non-missing data points, rather than the total sample size, were taken as the base, but this can be very confusing to the reader. It is best to include "missing" as an extra category.

Reference was just made to the base on which percentages are calculated. That brings me to the second caution to be observed. Be careful of the changing base. There is an old joke about an employee who had to take a 50% decrease in salary from $400 a week to $200 a week, which the boss "restored" a month later by giving him a 50% increase. Because of the change in the base he wound up at only $300 a week, not at the original $400. In research, a common problem is that the investigator might try to compare the percentage of a *total* group at Time 1 to the percentage of the *surviving* group at Time 2. Suppose that in a longitudinal study of a particular birth cohort of elderly people (say a group of people born in 1900), 5% had Alzheimer's disease at 80 years of age but only 1% had Alzheimer's disease at 90 years of age. That does not mean that the cohort got better. The base at age 80 may have been 1,000 and the base at age 90 may have been 700, with 43 of the original 50 Alzheimer's patients having died between age 80 and age 90.

A third caution concerns the way in which you do the percentaging. If you want to study the relationship between something like religious preference (the independent variable) and health status (the dependent variable), then you compare, for example, the percentage of Christians who are reported to be in good health to the percentage of non-Christians who are reported to be in good health; you do *not* compare the percentage of those in good health who are Christians to the percentage of those in bad health who are Christians.

A fourth caution has to do with the making of more than one comparison with percentages that have to add to 100. For example, if there is a difference of 30% between the percentage of Christians in good health and the percentage of non-Christians in good health, then there must be a compensating difference in the opposite direction between the percentage of Christians in bad health and the percentage of non-Christians in bad health. A similar caution has to do with claims such as "80% of Christians are in good health, whereas only 20% are in bad health." If 80% are in good health, then of course 20% are in non-good (i.e., bad) health.

A fifth caution concerns very small bases. Percentages are both unnecessary and misleading when they are based on small sample sizes. (It goes without saying, but I will say it anyhow, that the base *always* should be provided.) If 80% of Christians are reported to be in good health and 50% of non-Christians are reported to be in good health, then that is no big deal if there are just 10 Christians and 10 non-Christians in the total sample because that is a difference of only three people.

Believe it or not, there are some very good quantitative nursing research studies for which the principal statistical analyses employed are simple percentage calculations. For two interesting examples of such studies, see Brown, Arnold, Allison, Klein, and Jacobsen (1993) and Pollow, Stoller, Forster, and Duniho (1994).

DESCRIPTIVE STATISTICS

There are two general types of statistics: descriptive and inferential. Descriptive statistics are discussed in the next three sections, and inferential statistics are treated in the subsequent sections.

Frequency Distributions

As the term implies, **descriptive statistics** are ways of summarizing the principal features of the data you happen to have. Consider the hypothetical data in Table 11.1 for four of the variables used as prototypical examples of different levels of measurement in Chapter 10. (Note that the same numerals [1, 2, 3, and 4] are used for all four variables.) Suppose that these data were obtained for a simple random sample of 64 premature infants drawn from a very large population of premature infants at a metropolitan hospital, with information provided at time of delivery on parent's religious affiliation ("religion"), infant's health status ("health"), infant's body

Table 11.1 Some Data

Person	Religion	Health	Temperature	Weight
1	1	4	3	3
2	4	1	3	4
3	3	2	1	4
4	4	3	4	2
5	1	1	3	3
6	3	4	3	2
7	3	3	4	1
8	3	3	3	2
9	2	3	4	1
10	1	1	2	4
11	3	2	2	4
12	4	4	4	1
13	3	1	2	4
14	3	3	3	3
15	3	1	3	3
16	3	2	3	2
17	1	1	1	4
18	3	4	3	3
19	4	2	4	3
20	3	2	3	3
21	3	1	1	4
22	1	2	1	4
23	3	1	1	4
24	3	4	4	1
25	4	4	2	3
26	3	3	1	4
27	3	2	2	3
28	2	1	1	4
29	1	3	3	3
30	2	2	2	3
31	3	2	4	1
32	3	3	2	4
33	2	1	2	4
34	3	1	4	1
35	3	2	3	2
36	4	3	2	4
37	4	3	3	3

(continued)

Table 11.1 Continued

Person	Religion	Health	Temperature	Weight
38	1	2	2	4
39	1	1	3	2
40	3	1	3	3
41	3	1	3	2
42	1	4	1	4
43	3	1	3	2
44	1	1	4	1
45	1	2	3	3
46	3	1	4	1
47	3	2	4	1
48	1	4	4	1
49	1	3	3	2
50	3	1	2	4
51	1	3	4	1
52	3	2	2	4
53	4	2	3	3
54	3	2	1	4
55	1	2	3	2
56	1	2	4	1
57	3	4	2	4
58	4	4	3	3
59	1	4	3	2
60	1	3	1	4
61	3	4	1	4
62	1	4	2	4
63	2	3	3	2
64	1	3	2	4

NOTE: Scoring is as follows. Religion: 1 = Protestant, 2 = Catholic, 3 = Jewish, 4 = other or none; Health: 1 = good, 2 = stable, 3 = guarded, 4 = critical; Temperature: number of degrees above the "normal" 99°; Weight: number of pounds.

temperature ("temperature"), and infant's body weight ("weight"), which are nominal, ordinal, interval, and ratio variables, respectively.

One of the first things to do with such data is to prepare a **frequency distribution** for each of the variables, which gives a count of the number and/or percentage of infants in each category of each variable. An example of a frequency distribution for the health variable is provided in Table 11.2. This distribution is a vast improvement over the long list of scores for that

Table 11.2 A Frequency Distribution for the "Health" Variable ($N = 64$)

Health	Tally	Frequency	Percentage[a]
1 (good)	111111111111111111	18	28.1
2 (stable)	111111111111111111	18	28.1
3 (guarded)	111111111111111	15	23.4
4 (critical)	1111111111111	13	20.3

a. The percentages do not add to exactly 100 due to rounding.

variable in the third column of Table 11.1. (I use the word "scores" generically to refer to any set of measurements on any variable, even if the context has nothing to do with scores in the educational testing sense.) As indicated in Table 11.2, the health status of 18 of the infants (28.1%) was reported to be "good," another 18 were reported to be "stable," 15 (23.4%) were in "guarded" condition, and 13 (20.3%) were "critical." The percentages add to 99.9 rather than 100 because of rounding.

Cross-Tabulations

It is the rare research question, however, that is concerned merely with counts or percentages for a single variable. Most research questions involve *relationships between two variables.* (Recall some of the questions in Chapters 3 and 7. Does smoking cause lung cancer? Does obesity contribute to the incidence of coronary disease?)

Suppose that a researcher was interested in the relationship between parent's religious affiliation and infant's health status for this sample of 64 babies. (Do not ask me why anybody might be interested in that relationship, but the decision of what question to ask *always* should be the researcher's choice and no one else's.) The appropriate way in which to investigate the relationship between two nominal variables, between two ordinal variables, or between one nominal variable and one ordinal variable (the actual case here) is to set up a two-way frequency distribution called a **cross-tabulation** or **contingency table**. The cross-tabulation of the religion and health variables is displayed in Table 11.3. That table contains a wealth of descriptive information regarding the relationship between the two variables such as the following:

Table 11.3 A Cross-Tabulation (contingency table) for the "Religion" and "Health" Variables

| Health | Religion | | | | Total |
	1 (Protestant)	*2 (Catholic)*	*3 (Jewish)*	*4 (other/none)*	*Total*
1 (good)	5 (25)	2 (40)	10 (33.3)	1 (11.1)	18
2 (stable)	5 (25)	1 (20)	10 (33.3)	2 (22.2)	18
3 (guarded)	5 (25)	2 (40)	5 (16.7)	3 (33.3)	15
4 (critical)	5 (25)	0 (0)	5 (16.7)	3 (33.3)	13
Total	20	5	30	9	64

NOTE: Percentages are in parentheses. Some do not add exactly to 100 due to rounding.

1. For the 20 Protestants, 5 of their babies were rated to be in good condition, 5 stable, 5 guarded, and 5 critical. This information, all by itself, begins to suggest that there is very little, if any, relationship between the two variables.

2. Among the sample, 5 out of 20 (25%) Protestant babies, 2 out of 5 (40%) Catholic babies, 10 out of 30 (33.3%) Jewish babies, and 1 out of 9 (11.1%) babies in the "other" or "none" categories were rated to be in good condition. Because those four percentages are not widely different from one another, that information further suggests that there is not a very strong relationship between religious preference and health status.

3. The row and column totals, called *marginals,* give us frequency distributions for each of the variables taken separately "for free." (Compare the data for the health variable to the corresponding data in Table 11.2.)

Note especially the way in which the percentaging is done. The usual conventions are to take as the column headings the categories of the independent variable and take as the row headings the categories of the dependent variable, to percentage down the columns, and to compare those percentages across the rows (see Elifson, Runyon, & Haber, 1982). For this example, religious preference is the independent variable and health status is the dependent variable. Religious affiliation of parent is a possible, albeit unlikely, cause of infant health status; it would make less sense to take health status of the infants as a possible cause of religious affiliation of their parents. In neither case, however, can causality be demonstrated given that the three criteria necessary to establish cause-and-effect relationships (see Chapter 3) cannot be satisfied by these data.

In the second point in the preceding list, a comparison of the 25%, 40%, 33.3%, and 11.1% for the first row of the contingency table already has been made. For the remaining rows, the corresponding figures are 25%, 20%, 33.3%, 22.2% (second row); 25%, 40%, 16.7%, 33.3% (third row); and 25%, 0%, 16.7%, 33.3% (fourth row). Those also are fairly close to one another, further reinforcing the absence of a very strong relationship between the two variables.

There are two problems with this cross-tabulation, however. The first is that the data still require further summarization because it would be very difficult to keep track of all those various counts and percentages. There is a statistic called a **contingency coefficient** (naturally enough), which takes on a value of 0 if there is absolutely no relationship whatsoever between two variables and which takes on a value close to 1 if there is a perfect relationship. It can take on any value between those two numbers, and for real data it rarely will be equal to either of the end points. For the data in Table 11.3, the contingency coefficient turns out to be .29, which indicates some, but not much, relationship between the religion and health variables for these 64 infants.

The other problem is that there are too many "cells" in this table (each box in the table is called a cell) for a sample of only 64 subjects. With 16 cells and 64 subjects, there is an average of only 4 subjects per cell, and that is not enough to get a good feel for the data. What often is suggested when this happens is to combine certain categories and recompute the various statistics. I have done this for the religion variable by combining Protestants with Catholics (calling them "Christians") and by combining Jewish with the "other" and "none" categories to create a "non-Christian" category. For the health variable, I combined the good and stable statuses (calling them "satisfactory") and combined the guarded and critical statuses ("unsatisfactory"). The resulting 2 × 2 cross-tabulation is shown in Table 11.4, and the contingency coefficient for this table is .07, which is even less than the calculated value for Table 11.3. (That often happens.)

Scatter Plots

For two interval variables, two ratio variables, or one interval variable and one ratio variable, relationships usually are explored through the use of traditional two-dimensional geometrical data plots, often called **scatter plots** or **scatter diagrams**, rather than by preparing cross-tabulations. (For

Table 11.4 Revised Cross-Tabulation for "Religion" and "Health" Variables

| | Religion | | |
Health	1 (Christian)	0 (non-Christian)	Total
1 (satisfactory)	13 (52.0)	23 (59.0)	36
0 (unsatisfactory)	12 (48.0)	16 (41.0)	28
Total	25	39	64

NOTE: Percentages are in parentheses.

the remaining combinations, such as one ordinal variable and one ratio variable, consult your local friendly statistician!) In studying the relationship between body temperature (interval) and body weight (ratio) for our 64 hypothetical premature infants, we would take the data in Table 11.1 (the last two columns) and plot the weight variable on the vertical (y) axis against the temperature variable on the horizontal (x) axis or the other way around. The usual convention is to use y for the dependent variable and x for the independent variable. Figure 11.1 illustrates such a plot.

There appears to be a very strong relationship between weight and temperature, but it is in an inverse direction; that is, low temperatures (those very close to normal) tend to be associated with high weights, and high temperatures tend to be associated with low weights. But there still remains the problem of further summarization of the data. It would be nice to have a statistic similar to the contingency coefficient that would capture both the direction and magnitude of the relationship between two such variables. Fortunately, there is such a statistic, called the **Pearson product-moment correlation coefficient** or Pearson r for short. (I will not go into why it is called that.) It takes on a value of 0 for no relationship (just as the contingency coefficient does), a value of 1 for a perfect positive relationship (low goes with low and high goes with high), a value of –1 for a perfect negative relationship (low goes with high and high goes with low), or any other number between –1 and 1. For our data, the Pearson r is –.87, which is very close to –1 and, therefore, is indicative of a strong inverse relationship.

When investigating the relationship between two interval or ratio variables, it also is conventional to report various other statistics for the variables taken separately such as the average (technically called the *arithmetic mean*) and the *standard deviation* (a measure of the amount of variability in the data). The arithmetic mean is found by adding up all the

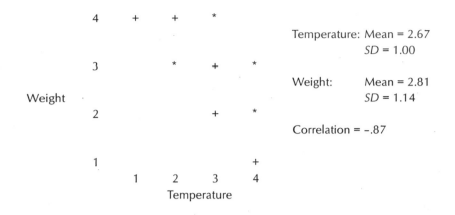

Figure 11.1. A Scatter Plot

NOTE: An asterisk (*) represents a single data point. A plus (+) sign represents more than one data point superimposed on one another. (There are actually 64 data points in all.) The mean for each of the two variables is the familiar average. The *SD* is the standard deviation and is an indication of the amount of variability in the data.

scores for a variable and dividing by the number of scores. The calculation of the standard deviation is considerably more complicated. The difference of each score from the mean is squared, those squared differences are averaged (producing a statistic called the *variance*), and the square root of the average squared difference is extracted. The arithmetic mean and the standard deviation for the temperature and weight variables are included in Figure 11.1.

The usual caution is in order for this example. The very high (although inverse) correlation tells you nothing about causality. The infants' high temperatures may or may not have "caused" their weights to be low, and the infants' low temperatures may or may not have "caused" their high body weights.

I must point out that the Pearson *r* is really only appropriate for describing the direction and magnitude of a *linear* relationship. If the data plot takes on a curvilinear pattern (e.g., something that resembles a U-shaped parabola), then you might want to abandon any further interest in Pearson *r* (and, once again, consult your local friendly statistician). A good rule to remember is to *always* plot the data before calculating Pearson *r* (or, better yet, have a computer do it for you).

INFERENTIAL STATISTICS

For full population data and nonrandom sample data, descriptive statistics are all you need and all you are justified in using (Barhyte, Redman, & Neill, 1990). But whenever you have drawn a random sample from a population and you are interested in generalizing from that sample to the population from which it was drawn, you invariably will use inferential statistics as the basis for such a generalization. (The situation is actually more complicated and controversial than the last two sentences suggest. There are those who use inferential statistics *whether or not* their sample is random and sometimes even when they have full population data, using as a rationale an argument that goes something like this: "I know I did not draw the subjects at random, but I would like to generalize to a hypothetical population of subjects *like these.*")

Parameters and Statistics

Inferential statistics are procedures for either estimating a **parameter** for a population or testing a hypothesis concerning a parameter. Although the term has other meanings in science, in the context of inferential statistics a parameter is a summary index for a population such as a population mean (average), a population standard deviation, or a population correlation coefficient. Here is how inferential statistics works. First, you calculate a descriptive **statistic** for your sample such as a sample mean, a sample standard deviation, or a sample correlation coefficient. Then either you estimate the corresponding population parameter by putting some sort of "confidence (tolerance) limits" around that sample statistic (the process is called **interval estimation**) or you use the sample statistic to test some hypothesized value for the corresponding population parameter (that approach is called, naturally enough, **hypothesis testing**). For example, you might have a sample correlation coefficient (Pearson *r*) of .50 and you apply the appropriate formulas to estimate that the population correlation coefficient is a number somewhere between .25 and .70. Or, you might use that same statistic of .50 to test the hypothesis that the population correlation coefficient is equal to 0, and by applying slight variations of the same formulas, you reject that hypothesis. In nursing research, the testing of hypotheses about parameters is far more commonly encountered than is estimating them. But in some other sciences, interval estimation is preferred. In psychology, for example, at the time of the writing of this chapter (mid-1997), there is a task force that is considering a recommendation to do away with hypothesis testing entirely and to replace it with interval estimation for individual studies and with meta-analysis (see Chapter 14) for pooling results across studies. One of the arguments for the exclusive use of interval estimation is that you often can get hypothesis testing for free. (If the hypothesized parameter is inside the interval, then it cannot be rejected; if it is not inside the interval, then it can be rejected.)

Hypothesis Testing (Significance Testing)

There are two types of hypothesis-testing procedures: (a) **parametric tests** (e.g., the *t* test), for which a number of assumptions need to be made about the population from which the sample(s) has (have) been drawn (e.g., that the distribution of the variable in the population is of the normal, or "bell-shaped," form); and (b) **nonparametric tests** (e.g., the Mann-Whitney *U* test), for which few or no assumptions need to be made. There is a common confusion in some of the nursing research literature regarding the distinction between parametric and nonparametric tests. Some authors claim that parametric tests are used for large samples and that nonparametric tests are used for small samples. That is not the basis for the distinction; sample size has nothing to do with it. Some other authors argue that parametric statistics are used to make inferences from samples to populations and that nonparametric statistics are used to describe samples. That also is not true; both are inferential, not descriptive, statistics. Figure 11.2 should help clarify the situation.

Two of the most commonly encountered hypothesis-testing procedures are the **chi-square test** and the *t* **test**. Although I do not discuss the formulas for these tests here (those who are interested are referred to the various sources listed near the end of this chapter), I include an example of each.

Consider the two relationship questions considered in the descriptive statistics section of this chapter, namely the relationship between religious affiliation and health status and the relationship between body temperature and body weight. By applying a chi-square test to the cross-tabulated data in Table 11.4, the hypothesis that there is no relationship between the religion and health variables in the premature infant population cannot be rejected because the sample statistic of .07 could easily be obtained by

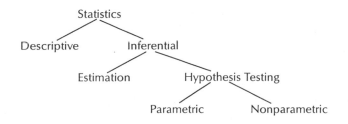

Figure 11.2. Types of Statistics

chance in a sample of 64 infants even if the corresponding population parameter is equal to 0.

For the relationship between the temperature and weight variables, on the other hand, application of a *t* test for Pearson's *r* would reject the hypothesis that there is no relationship between these two variables in the population because the difference between the sample statistic of –.87 and the hypothesized parameter of 0 is unlikely to be attributed to chance. (Whenever the so-called **null hypothesis** of no relationship between two variables is rejected, the sample result is said to be **statistically significant**.)

Regarding the *t* test, in the quantitative literature, the *t* test usually is associated with a test of the significance of the difference between two *means*. It turns out that it also can be used to test the significance of a correlation coefficient (see, e.g., Tatsuoka, 1993).

Statistical Significance Versus Practical Importance

It is essential to understand that statistical significance is not the same as practical (clinical) importance (Oberst, 1982; LeFort, 1992; Kirk, 1996; for an example, see Baker, Bidwell-Cerone, Gaze, & Knapp, 1984). If the sample size is large enough, even the tiniest relationship can be statistically significant. Statistical significance also is not the same thing as proof. We cannot prove that the null hypothesis is true, nor can we prove that it is false. (The only science in which proof is attainable is mathematics.) All we can do is determine whether the data support the null hypothesis or whether the data do not support the null hypothesis.

There is a great deal of additional jargon associated with various hypothesis-testing procedures such as degrees of freedom, Type I and Type II errors, and one-tailed and two-tailed tests, but because this is not a statistics text, I cannot go into all of the details that would be necessary to understand such matters. I should point out, however, that there is an interesting connection between Type I and Type II errors and the notions of "false positives" and "false negatives" alluded to in Chapter 10. The making of a Type I error (rejecting a true null hypothesis) in a statistical inference is analogous to making a false positive judgment that a person has a particular disease when in fact the person does not have the disease. Similarly, the making of a Type II error (not rejecting a false null hypothesisis) is analogous to the false negative judgment that a person does not have a disease when in fact the person does.

Regression Analysis

One type of statistical analysis that is used in virtually all the sciences is regression analysis, both descriptively and inferentially. **Regression analysis** is a technique that is closely associated with the scatter plots and the Pearson *r*'s referred to earlier and to "ordinary" correlational research in general. In addition to the "goodness" or "badness" of linear relationships indicated by Pearson *r*'s, regression analysis focuses on the coefficients in the **regression equation** that connect a dependent variable with one or more independent variables. Although the mathematical intricacies can get rather complicated, the basic concepts of regression analysis are actually very straightforward. It is to those concepts that I now turn.

First, it is well to distinguish between "simple" regression analysis (one dependent variable and one independent variable) and **multiple regression analysis** (one dependent variable and two or more independent variables). The objective of simple regression analysis is to find the **slope** and **intercept** of the equation of the line that "best fits" the data when the measures for the dependent variable are plotted on the vertical (*Y*) axis against the measures for the independent variable on the horizontal (*X*) axis. (See the earlier discussion of scatter plots.) The slope of that best-fitting line is the increase (or decrease) in *Y* that is associated with a one-unit increase in *X*. (It is an increase for a positive relationship and a decrease for a negative relationship.) The intercept of the best-fitting line is the point at which the line crosses the *Y* axis and corresponds to the value of *Y* when *X* is equal to zero, which may or may not be a meaningful value.

For the weight versus temperature example considered earlier, the steep negative slope of the line is −.99 and the intercept is 5.45. For those data, therefore, for every 1° increase in temperature, there is an associated (not necessarily causally) decrease of .99 pound. The intercept of 5.45 for this example is not meaningful because a temperature of 0° is outside the range of possible values for X and 5.45 is outside the range of possible values for Y. This regression equation also could be used in predicting unknown values of Y for subsequent subjects for whom X is known. For example, it can be shown that a subject who had a temperature 3° above normal would be expected to have a weight of approximately 2.48 pounds.

It is multiple regression analysis, however, that is much more commonly encountered in nursing research. The reason is that it is very difficult to explore, predict, or explain a dependent variable by using only one independent variable. It makes sense, and the mathematics of the technique corroborate it, that a *combination* of carefully chosen independent variables should do a better job of "accounting for" (again, not necessarily causally) the dependent variable of direct concern. For two independent variables, for example, there are two "slopes" that can be determined, one for each independent variable. (The word "slopes" is enclosed in quotation marks here because it is the equation of the *plane* of best fit, rather than a line, that is sought, and a plane has two "tilts" rather than a single slope.) The "slope" for an independent variable in a multiple regression analysis is the amount of increase (or decrease) in the dependent variable that is associated with a one-unit increase in that independent variable, *statistically controlling for* (holding constant, partialling out, etc.) the other independent variable. The measure of goodness or badness of overall fit is the **multiple correlation coefficient**, which is the Pearson r between the dependent variable and the best linear combination of the two independent variables.

There is nothing special about two independent variables. Multiple regression analysis has been generalized to be used with any number of independent variables (within reason). Real-world applications sometimes have as many as 10 or 20 independent variables, but there tends to be a point of diminishing returns when the number of independent variables exceeds 5 or 6.

You will find in the literature that there are actually three types of multiple regression analyses. The first type is called **simultaneous regression**. This is the simplest and most commonly encountered type. In simultaneous regression, all of the independent variables are "entered" at the same time in a single analysis with the contribution of each assessed while statistically controlling for the others. The second type is called **hierarchical regression.** This is the most useful for explanatory purposes in attempting to determine the "effect" (not necessarily causal) of one or more independent variables *over and above* the "effect" (again, not necessarily causal) of one or more other independent variables (often called **covariates**) that need to be statistically controlled. The covariates are entered first, and the variables of principal concern are entered last. The third type is called **stepwise regression.** This often is confused with hierarchical regression in that the independent variables are entered sequentially rather than simultaneously, but there is a very important difference between hierarchical regression and stepwise regression. In hierarchical regression, the entry of the independent variables is based on theoretical considerations and is completely under the control of the researcher. In stepwise regression, entry (or non-entry) is determined entirely on the basis of statistical significance. Because of this, and for some other technical reasons, stepwise regression usually is regarded as an inferior approach and should generally be avoided (Aaronson, 1989). I believe that hierarchical regression analysis is the most useful type of regression analysis for most quantitative nursing research applications because we often are interested in the "effects" of certain variables over and above the "effects" of others. (For a good example, see Pender, Walker, Sechrist, & Frank-Stromborg, 1990.)

If the dependent variable is dichotomous (two nominal categories), then multiple regression analysis is not appropriate and a related technique, **logistic regression analysis,** should be used. (For examples, see Hall & Farel, 1988; Jones, 1992; Lauver, Nabholz, Scott, & Tak, 1997; Long & Boik, 1993; Menard, 1995; Palmer, German, & Ouslander, 1991; and Yarandi & Simpson, 1991.) If there is more than one dependent variable, no matter their types, some sort of *multivariate analysis* is required. (For details, see Harris, 1985; Marascuilo & Levin, 1983; and Tabachnick & Fidell, 1996.)

Some Applications of
Regression Analysis to Nursing Research

Just about every issue of *Nursing Research* and *Research in Nursing & Health* has at least one article that includes regression statistics in the analysis of the research data (see, e.g., Logsdon, McBride, & Birkimer, 1994). Unfortunately, the information that is provided varies considerably from one research report to another. As evidence of this and for typical illustrations of the use of regression analysis in quantitative nursing research, see the examples that were cited previously in Chapter 7 in the section on "ordinary" predictive correlational studies (Koniak-Griffin & Brecht, 1995; Munro, 1985; Schraeder, 1986). I have tried to remedy the chaotic situation regarding the reporting of regression results (Knapp, 1994a). In a recent study that applied regression analysis to nursing research, Brown, Knapp, and Radke (1997) provided examples of what we believe to be the essential information for the proper interpretation of the results of regression analyses.

Path Analysis, Structural Equation Modeling, and Their Applications to Nursing Research

For the "explanatory" type of correlational research, path analysis is the most common method for testing how well a hypothesized model fits empirical data. Consider the simple **path model** depicted in the (a) part of Figure 11.3. It hypothesizes that stress has a direct "effect" (not necessarily causal) on depression. The plus (+) sign placed on the arrow postulates a positive relationship (as stress increases, depression increases). To test that hypothesis, a researcher has essentially two choices; he or she can either (a) perform an experiment in which stress is manipulated (the experimental group gets stressed and the control group does not) and see what happens to depression or (b) measure both stress and depression with available inventories and see what the direction and strength of the relationship are between score on the stress scale and score on the depression scale. (The latter choice is likely to be the preferred one because the former creates ethical problems associated with the artificial assignment of human subjects to stressful situations.) Simple regression analysis (one X and one Y) can be used to analyze the data in either event. Support for the model would be provided by a positive slope. In this context, the slopes are called **path coefficients.**

Now consider the more complicated model in the (b) part of Figure 11.3. It hypothesizes that stress has both a **direct "effect"** on depression and an **indirect "effect"** (through social support, perhaps loss of social support) on depression, with neither effect necessarily causal. The plus (+) sign on the

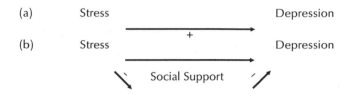

Figure 11.3. Two Models for the "Effect" of Stress on Depression

arrow from stress to depression postulates a positive relationship, as before; the minus (–) sign on the arrow from stress to social support postulates a negative relationship (as stress increases, social support decreases); and the minus (–) sign on the arrow from social support to depression also postulates a negative relationship between those two constructs (as social support increases, depression decreases). Again the researcher has the experimental and nonexperimental options for designing a study that would test this model (with the preference likely to be given to the nonexperimental approach), and regression can be used for the analysis of the data. But this time *two* regression analyses are required: (a) a simple regression analysis with social support as the dependent variable and with stress as the independent variable and (b) a multiple regression analysis with depression as the dependent variable and with stress and social support as the independent variables. Support for Model (b) would be provided by a negative path coefficient for the first regression and by one positive and one negative path coefficient for the second regression (positive for the top path and negative for the lower right path). A measure of the indirect "effect" of stress on depression can be obtained by multiplying the lower left path coefficient by the lower right path coefficient. (For the details regarding this matter and other technical matters associated with **path analysis,** see Munro & Sexton, 1984, and Munro, 1997.)

Note that if the top path coefficient for testing Model (b) in Figure 11.3 is positive and either the lower left *or* lower right path coefficient is equal to zero, then Model (b) essentially reduces to Model (a). One of the more interesting applications of path analysis is to the *comparison* of *two* models for better fit to data. If simpler models such as Model (a) provide better fit than, or even approximately equal fit to, more complicated models such as Model (b), then scientific parsimony has been better accomplished.

It turns out that most real-life applications of path analysis to nursing research are for the testing of models that are even more complicated than Model (b) in Figure 11.3. For an interesting example of such models, see Lucas, Atwood, and Hagaman (1993) and my critique of that article (Knapp, 1994a). For other examples, see Acorn, Ratner, and Crawford (1997); Anderson (1995); Coffman, Levitt, and Brown (1994); Hall, Kotch, Browne, and Rayens (1996); Hanson (1997); Leveck and Jones (1996); Pohl, Boyd, Liang, and Given (1995); Smyth and Yarandi (1992); Wambach (1997); Weaver, Richmond, and Narsavage (1997); Wineman (1990); and Winslow (1997). The Hanson (1997) article is tricky; the model initially proposed was nonrecursive (bidirectional causality), but the model actually tested was recursive (unidirectional causality). The Weaver et al. (1997) article provides an interesting reformulation of a research problem addressed in a less sophisticated fashion by Weaver and Narsavage (1992).

An example of a study that was concerned with both direct and indirect effects, yet did *not* use path analysis, is the research reported by Yarcheski, Scoloveno, and Mahon (1994) on hopefulness as a mediating variable (see Chapter 3) regarding the relationship between social support and well-being.

Structural equation modeling (sometimes called covariance structure modeling or the analysis of covariance structures) extends path analysis further by incorporating into the model(s) to be tested "unmeasured" constructs as well as "measured" constructs and allows for the testing of reciprocal relationships (double-headed arrows) in addition to, or instead of, unidirectional relationships. Needless to say, things can get out of hand very quickly, despite readily available computer programs such as LISREL, EQS, and RAMONA. For the methodological details, see Boyd, Frey, and Aaronson (1988); Aaronson, Frey, and Boyd (1988); Mason-Hawkes and Holm (1989); and Munro (1997). For recent examples of the application of structural equation modeling to nursing research, see Bottorff, Johnson, Ratner, and Hayduk (1996); DeMaio-Esteves (1990); DiIorio, Hennessy, and Manteuffel (1996); Gurney, Mueller, and Price (1997); Johnson, Ratner, Bottorff, and Hayduk (1993); and Ratner, Bottorff, Johnson, and Hayduk (1994, 1996). The article by Ratner et al. (1994) is particularly noteworthy in that it described how one can test interaction effects within a structural equation model.

The March-April 1997 issue of *Nursing Research* contained three articles that reported the use of structural equation modeling (Carruth, Tate, Moffett, & Hill, 1997; Flynn, 1997; Yarcheski, Mahon, & Yarcheski, 1997). Interestingly, however, all were actually path analyses "run" as special cases of structural equation modeling because there were single indicators of all constructs and all the models were recursive.

ASSUMPTIONS

All statistical techniques have certain assumptions that should be satisfied if the techniques are to be used properly. Some of these assumptions are more important than others, and the prospective user often can appeal to the "robustness" of the technique with respect to minor violations of an assumption. A case in point is the assumption of a normal (bell-shaped) frequency distribution of the measurements in the population from which a sample has been randomly drawn. If the researcher has reason to believe that the population distribution is not too badly skewed, then the procedure probably can be employed without serious consequences. But you cannot overdo it. If the dependent variable of interest is something like income, which is very non-normally distributed in just about every population, then you are advised to entertain some sort of data transformation to better satisfy the normal assumption. (For details regarding data transformations in general, see Ferketich & Verran, 1994.)

THE "CRAFT" OF STATISTICS

Most people are under the impression that statistics is all science and no craft. That is not true. Those who are good at statistics have developed certain skills and insights that they have found to be particularly useful when applying statistical techniques to research problems. I now share some of their "secrets."

One of the skills that is nice to have is the ability to know how much data to include in a research report (Knapp, 1994a). Editors and reviewers of professional journals are constantly asking authors to add this analysis, delete that table, or some such request. The following guidelines should help:

1. Do not provide so much information about the subjects that the reader loses interest in the major findings of the study.

2. *Always* include the descriptive statistics on which an inferential test is based. This is particularly relevant for the statistical test called the analysis of variance (ANOVA). It is all too common to see in a journal article an ANOVA summary table that tells you that the means are significantly different from one another without providing the numerical values of those means.

3. Unless the sample size is very small or the editor specifically asks for them, do not include the actual raw data ("scores") despite the advantages of such data. (See the discussions of the article by Mayo, Horne, Summers, Pearson, & Helsabeck, 1996, in Chapters 5 and 15.)

4. Because a picture often is worth a thousand words, try to include the scatter plot if your study involves only two (interval or ratio) variables, but do not be surprised if the editor eliminates it because figures cost much more to print than does text.

A related skill is knowing how many decimal places to report. Just because computers provide 5- or 10-place accuracy, it does not necessarily follow that all of those digits should be included. Just 2 or 3 digits to the right of the decimal point are plenty; any greater accuracy probably is not warranted by the data. One of the most serious (and, alas, most common) errors is to report a sample result as being significant at, say, the $p = .0000$ level. There are at least two things wrong with this: (a) that is too many decimal places and (b) there usually is no such thing as a zero probability of having occurred by chance; the actual p value has been rounded to .0000, which means less than .0001. (For more on the use and misuse of p values, see Slakter, Wu, & Suzuki-Slakter, 1991.)

A third bit of wisdom is knowing how little or how much to emphasize statistical significance. I already pointed out earlier in this chapter that significance testing is irrelevant for full populations and for nonrandom samples (although you would not know that from reading the literature). But even when the reporting of statistical significance is warranted, it should not be overdone. No more than a small percentage of the text of a research report should be devoted to the statistical significance (or lack of same) of the findings.

As a final tip, do not worry about insulting the reader's intelligence. Most people who read research journals would much rather have the analysis of the data be made simple to understand than to be the object of a "snow job" involving all types of fancy statistical jargon that they cannot comprehend.

RECOMMENDED READING

Here is a list of some books and articles that deal nicely with statistics:

1. Boyd, Frey, and Aaronson (1988) and Aaronson, Frey, and Boyd (1988): This set of articles explains the basic concepts involved in structural equation modeling.
2. Cohen (1988): This is a handy reference book that contains the tables that are helpful for determining the appropriate sample size for a given hypothesis-testing situation (see Chapter 9).
3. Darlington (1990): This is one of the best textbooks for regression analysis and related techniques.
4. Ferketich and Verran (1986) and Verran and Ferketich (1987a, 1987b): This is a series of three articles that provides nursing researchers with an excellent summary of the methods of "exploratory data analysis," a collection of unusual but useful ways of describing data, developed originally by Tukey (1977).
5. Knapp (1996a): This little book of mine explains basic statistical concepts by using an ordinary deck of playing cards.
6. Marcus-Roberts and Roberts (1987): This superb article contains the best discussion I have seen regarding why traditional statistical procedures (means, *t* tests, etc.) are inappropriate for ordinal scales.
7. McLaughlin and Marascuilo (1990): This is a recent statistics text for nursing research that applies a variety of statistical techniques to a hypothetical, but nevertheless very interesting, data set.
8. Munro (1997): This is a statistics text that is particularly good for explaining the principles of *path analysis* and *structural equation modeling* techniques, which currently are very popular in nursing research concerned with model testing.
9. Polit (1996): This is one of the most recent texts intended for nursing researchers, written by the first author of the popular research methods books.
10. Siegel and Castellan (1988): This is a revision of a very old, but very popular, textbook that discusses various nonparametric statistical techniques.

REFERENCES

Aaronson, L. S. (1989). A cautionary note on the use of stepwise regression. *Nursing Research, 38,* 309-311.

Aaronson, L. S., Frey, M. A., & Boyd, C. J. (1988). Structural equation models and nursing research: Part II. *Nursing Research, 37,* 315-317.

Acorn, S., Ratner, P. A., & Crawford, M. (1997). Decentralization as a determinant of autonomy, job satisfaction, and organizational commitment among nurse managers. *Nursing Research, 46,* 52-58.

Anderson, K. L. (1995). The effect of chronic obstructive pulmonary disease on quality of life. *Research in Nursing & Health, 18,* 547-556.

Baker, N. C., Bidwell-Cerone, S., Gaze, N., & Knapp, T. R. (1984). The effect of type of thermometer and length of time inserted on oral temperature measurements of afebrile subjects. *Nursing Research, 33,* 109-111.

Barhyte, D. Y., Redman, B. K., & Neill, K. M. (1990). Population or sample: Design decision. *Nursing Research, 39,* 309-310.

Bottorff, J. L., Johnson, J. L., Ratner, P. A., & Hayduk, L. A. (1996). The effects of cognitive-perceptual factors on health promotion behavior maintenance. *Nursing Research, 45,* 30-36.

Boyd, C. J., Frey, M. A., & Aaronson, L. S. (1988). Structural equation models and nursing research: Part I. *Nursing Research, 37,* 249-252.

Brown, J. K., Knapp, T. R., & Radke, K. J. (1997). Sex, age, height, and weight as predictors of selected physiologic outcomes. *Nursing Research, 46,* 101-104.

Brown, L. P., Arnold, L., Allison, D., Klein, M. E., & Jacobsen, B. (1993). Incidence and pattern of jaundice in healthy breast-fed infants during the first month of life. *Nursing Research, 42,* 106-110.

Carruth, A. K., Tate, U. S., Moffett, B. S., & Hill, K. (1997). Reciprocity, emotional well-being, and family functioning as determinants of family satisfaction in caregivers of elderly patients. *Nursing Research, 46,* 93-100.

Coffman, S., Levitt, M. J., & Brown, L. (1994). Effects of clarification of support expectations in prenatal couples. *Nursing Research, 43,* 111-116.

Cohen, J. (1988). *Statistical power analysis for the behavioral sciences* (2nd ed.). Hillsdale, NJ: Lawrence Erlbaum.

Darlington, R. B. (1990). *Regression and linear models.* New York: McGraw-Hill.

DeMaio-Esteves, M. (1990). Mediators of daily stress and perceived health status in adolescent girls. *Nursing Research, 39,* 360-364.

DiIorio, C., Hennessy, M., & Manteuffel, B. (1996). Epilepsy self-management: A test of a theoretical model. *Nursing Research, 45,* 211-217.

Elifson, K. W., Runyon, R. P., & Haber, A. (1982). *Fundamentals of social statistics.* Reading, MA: Addison-Wesley.

Ferketich, S. L., & Verran, J. (1986). Exploratory data analysis: Introduction. *Western Journal of Nursing Research, 8,* 464-466.

Ferketich, S. L., & Verran, J. (1994). An overview of data transformation. *Research in Nursing & Health, 17,* 393-396.

Flynn, L. (1997). The health practices of homeless women: A causal model. *Nursing Research, 46,* 72-77.

Gurney, C. A., Mueller, C. W., & Price, J. L. (1997). Job satisfaction and organizational attachment of nurses holding doctoral degrees. *Nursing Research, 46,* 163-171.

Hall, L. A., & Farel, A. M. (1988). Maternal stresses and depressive symptoms: Correlates of behavior problems in young children. *Nursing Research, 37,* 156-161.

Hall, L. A., Kotch, J. B., Browne, D. C., & Rayens, M. K. (1996). Self-esteem as a mediator of the effects of stress and social resources on depressive symptoms in postpartum mothers. *Nursing Research, 45,* 231-238.

Hanson, M. J. S. (1997). The theory of planned behavior applied to cigarette smoking in African-American, Puerto Rican, and non-Hispanic white teenage families. *Nursing Research, 46,* 155-162.

Harris, R. J. (1985). *A primer of multivariate statistics* (2nd ed.). New York: Academic Press.

Johnson, J. L., Ratner, P. A., Bottorff, J. L., & Hayduk, L. A. (1993). An exploration of Pender's Health Promotion Model using LISREL. *Nursing Research, 42,* 132-138.

Jones, K. R. (1992). Risk of hospitalization for chronic hemodialysis patients. *Image, 24,* 88-94.

Kirk, R. E. (1996). Practical significance: A concept whose time has come. *Educational and Psychological Measurement, 56,* 746-759.

Knapp, T. R. (1994a). Regression analyses: What to report. *Nursing Research, 43,* 187-189.

Knapp, T. R. (1996a). *Learning statistics through playing cards.* Thousand Oaks, CA: Sage.

Koniak-Griffin, D., & Brecht, M.-L. (1995). Linkages between sexual risk taking, substance abuse, and AIDS knowledge among pregnant adolescents and young mothers. *Nursing Research, 44,* 340-346.

Lauver, D., Nabholz, S., Scott, K., & Tak, Y. (1997). Testing theoretical explanations of mammography use. *Nursing Research, 46,* 32-39.

LeFort, S. M. (1992). The statistical versus clinical significance debate. *Image, 25,* 57-62.

Leveck, M. L., & Jones, C. B. (1996). The nursing practice environment, staff retention, and quality of care. *Research in Nursing & Health, 19,* 331-343.

Logsdon, M. C., McBride, A. B., & Birkimer, J. C. (1994). Social support and postpartum depression. *Research in Nursing & Health, 17,* 449-457.

Long, K. A., & Boik, R. J. (1993). Predicting alcohol use in rural children: A longitudinal study. *Nursing Research, 42,* 79-86.

Lucas, M. D., Atwood, J. R., & Hagaman, R. (1993). Replication and validation of Anticipated Turnover Model for urban registered nurses. *Nursing Research, 42,* 29-35.

Marascuilo, L. A., & Levin, J. R. (1983). *Multivariate statistics in the social sciences.* Pacific Grove, CA: Brooks/Cole.

Marcus-Roberts, H., & Roberts, F. (1987). Meaningless statistics. *Journal of Educational Statistics, 12,* 383-394.

Mason-Hawkes, J., & Holm, K. (1989). Causal modeling: A comparison of path analysis and LISREL. *Nursing Research, 38,* 312-314.

Mayo, D. J., Horne, M. K., III, Summers, B. L., Pearson, D. C., & Helsabeck, C. B. (1996). The effects of heparin flush on patency of the Groshong catheter. *Oncology Nursing Forum, 23,* 1401-1405.

McLaughlin, F. E., & Marascuilo, L. A. (1990). *Advanced nursing and health care research: Quantification approaches.* Philadelphia: W. B. Saunders.

Menard, S. (1995). *Applied logistic regression analysis.* Thousand Oaks, CA: Sage.

Munro, B. H. (1985). Predicting success in graduate clinical specialty programs. *Nursing Research, 34,* 54-57.

Munro, B. H. (1997). *Statistics for health care research* (3rd ed.). Philadelphia: Lippincott.

Munro, B. H., & Sexton, D. L. (1984). Path analysis: A method for theory testing. *Western Journal of Nursing Research, 6,* 97-106.

Oberst, M. T. (1982). Clinical versus statistical significance. *Cancer Nursing, 5,* 475-476.

Palmer, M. H., German, P. S., & Ouslander, J. G. (1991). Risk factors for urinary incontinence one year after nursing home admission. *Research in Nursing & Health, 14,* 405-412.

Pender, N. J., Walker, S. N., Sechrist, K. R., & Frank-Stromborg, M. (1990). Predicting health-promoting lifestyles in the workplace. *Nursing Research, 39,* 326-332.

Pohl, J. M., Boyd, C., Liang, J., & Given, C. W. (1995). Analysis of the impact of mother-daughter relationships on the commitment to caregiving. *Nursing Research, 44,* 68-75.

Polit, D. F. (1996). *Data analysis and statistics for nursing research.* Stamford, CT: Appleton & Lange.

Pollow, R. L., Stoller, E. P., Forster, L. E., & Duniho, T. S. (1994). Drug combinations and potential for risk of adverse drug reaction among community-dwelling elderly. *Nursing Research, 43,* 44-49.

Ratner, P. A., Bottorff, J. L., Johnson, J. L., & Hayduk, L. A. (1994). The interaction effects of gender within the Health Promotion Model. *Research in Nursing & Health, 17,* 341-350.

Ratner, P. A., Bottorff, J. L., Johnson, J. L., & Hayduk, L. A. (1996). Using multiple indicators to test the dimensionality of concepts in the Health Promotion Model. *Research in Nursing & Health, 19,* 237-247.

Schraeder, B. D. (1986). Developmental progress in very low birth weight infants during the first year of life. *Nursing Research, 35,* 237-242.

Siegel, S., & Castellan, N. J. (1988). *Nonparametric statistics for the behavioral sciences* (2nd ed.). New York: McGraw-Hill.

Slakter, M. J., Wu, Y.-W. B., & Suzuki-Slakter, N. S. (1991). *, **, and ***: Statistical nonsense at the .00000 level. *Nursing Research, 40,* 248-249.

Smyth, K. A., & Yarandi, H. N. (1992). A path model of Type A and Type B responses to coping and stress in employed black women. *Nursing Research, 41,* 260-265.

Tabachnick, B. G., & Fidell, L. S. (1996). *Using multivariate statistics* (3rd ed.). New York: HarperCollins.

Tatsuoka, M. M. (1993). Elements of the general linear model. In G. Keren & C. Lewis (Eds.), *A handbook for data analysis in the behavioral sciences: Statistical issues* (pp. 3-41). Hillsdale, NJ: Lawrence Erlbaum.

Tukey, J. W. (1977). *Exploratory data analysis.* Reading, MA: Addison-Wesley.

Verran, J., & Ferketich, S. L. (1987a). Exploratory data analysis: Comparison of groups and variables. *Western Journal of Nursing Research, 9,* 617-625.

Verran, J., & Ferketich, S. L. (1987b). Exploratory data analysis: Examining single distributions. *Western Journal of Nursing Research, 9,* 142-149.

Wambach, K. A. (1997). Breastfeeding intention and outcome: A test of the theory of planned behavior. *Research in Nursing & Health, 20,* 51-59.

Weaver, T. E., & Narsavage, G. L. (1992). Physiological and psychological variables related to functional status in chronic obstructive lung disease. *Nursing Research, 41,* 286-291.

Weaver, T. E., Richmond, T. S., & Narsavage, G. L. (1997). An explanatory model of functional status in chronic obstructive pulmonary disease. *Nursing Research, 46,* 26-31.

Wineman, N. M. (1990). Adaptation to multiple sclerosis: The role of social support, functional disability, and perceived uncertainty. *Nursing Research, 39,* 294-299.

Winslow, B. W. (1997). Effects of formal supports on stress outcomes in family caregivers of Alzheimer's patients. *Research in Nursing & Health, 20,* 27-37.

Yarandi, H. N., & Simpson, S. H. (1991). The logistic regression model and the odds of testing HIV positive. *Nursing Research, 40,* 372-373.

Yarcheski, A., Mahon, N. E., & Yarcheski, T. J. (1997). Alternate models of positive health practices in adolescents. *Nursing Research, 46,* 85-92.

Yarcheski, A., Scoloveno, M. A., & Mahon, N. E. (1994). Social support and well-being in adolescents: The mediating role of hopefulness. *Nursing Research, 43,* 288-292.

STUDY SUGGESTIONS

1. For the article you chose for the study suggestion at the end of Chapter 9, identify each of the following:

a. The population of interest
b. The sample actually studied
c. The parameter(s) of principal concern
d. The descriptive statistic(s) reported
e. The inferential statistics used (if any)

2. Look up the study by Wineman (1990) that used path analysis and was cited in this chapter. See how much of it you can understand. (I think you will be pleasantly surprised.)

CHAPTER 12

The Use of Computers in Quantitative Research

CHAPTER OUTLINE

Key Terms: software, hardware

Some people like big ("mainframe") computers, some like small ("micro") computers or PCs (either Macintoshes or IBM-DOS machines and their various clones), and a few like in-between-size ("mini") computers. When it comes to choosing statistical "packages" for carrying out their data analyses, some people like SAS, some like SPSS, some like EXCEL, some like MINITAB (e.g., me) and other user-friendly packages, and some even like to write their own programs. The situation is equally chaotic so far as word processing is concerned. The manuscript for this text was prepared using WordPerfect, but any of a hundred or so different types of word processing **software** probably would have been just as good.

So, instead of trying to explain the different parts of a computer's **hardware** or showing examples of printouts of the results of analyses carried out using SAS or SPSS or whatever (Munro's [1997] text has some good examples of SPSS printouts), I concentrate in this chapter on some of the various ways in which computers have been and/or could be used in quantitative nursing research, and I include at the end of the chapter a few references for the reader who is interested in some of the more technical aspects of computers.

THE USE OF COMPUTERS WITHIN A TRADITIONAL QUANTITATIVE STUDY

One of the least common, but potentially most fruitful, ways in which computers are used in quantitative research is in the actual data-gathering process. Examples of such uses range from the rather straightforward recording of reaction times in psychological experiments ("Press the button when you see the light flash or hear the bell ring") to the entering of notes in observational studies. There are countless errors made in nursing investigations in transposing data from handwritten documents to more permanent records. Automating the data entry process helps considerably in reducing such errors.

A particularly creative illustration of the use of computers within an actual study was described by Holm (1981). In measuring husband-wife interactions, the observer used a handheld microprocessor unit to record her observations. These observations later were transferred electronically to a computer for subsequent data analysis.

Another example was provided by White, Wear, and Stephenson (1983), who recorded and analyzed the falling asleep behavior of 18 hospitalized children with something called the Senders Signals and Receivers Systems, a computer-compatible device consisting of a keyboard, an audio recorder, a playback tape deck, and a signal-conditioning circuit. This observational procedure also had been described in an earlier article by White and Wear (1980).

There also is a small amount of nursing research that studies the clinical use of computers, that is, the extent to which computers can be used in actual nursing care. A good example of such a study is the experiment carried out by Brennan, Moore, and Smyth (1991, 1995), who found that a computerized information network for caregivers of persons with Alzheimer's disease enhanced confidence in decision making about their loved ones but did not affect their actual decision-making skills. Another example is the research by Staggers and Mills (1994), who studied the relationship between various background characteristics of nurses and their computer skills.

THE USE OF COMPUTERS
FOR DATA ANALYSIS

This is far and away the most frequently encountered application of computers to quantitative investigations. Hardly anyone these days calculates a mean without using a computer, to say nothing of a complicated regression analysis or factor analysis. This is both a blessing and a tragedy. The obvious advantages of computerized analyses are speed, capacity, and accuracy. A regression analysis with, say, 10 independent variables and 100 subjects would take forever by hand, even if the analyst could keep track of all the data and never make any mistakes (both of which are essentially impossible). But the price that we pay for using such computerized analyses is *distancing* from our data. In turning the data over to an impersonal computer for "massaging," modern-day researchers rarely have the opportunity to get their hands dirty by exploring the data themselves. Too often overlooked are the unusual "outlier" or the truncated variable that can make the difference between a weak relationship and a strong one. (In fairness, there are computer subroutines that plot the data, tag potential outliers, warn about lack of variability, etc., but they almost never are used by nursing researchers.)

Computers also can be used for data entry, for data "cleaning" (correcting errors, etc.), and for various data transformations. Harrison (1989) described a procedure for connecting biological instrumentation directly to a computer for automatic entry of research data. Dennis (1994) discussed a technique for combining optical scanning with computers to manage data obtained through the use of questionnaires. Yarandi (1993) showed how readily available computer software (SAS) could be used to transform multicategoried nominal variables into a set of "dummy" variables for use in regression analyses.

Two other recent articles also addressed the use of computers for data entry. Both appeared in the "Practical Computer" section of the November-

December 1996 issue of *Nursing Research*. The first article, by Huang, Wilkie, and Berry (1996), discussed a procedure for both scoring and entering data for visual analog scales. The second article, by Davidson, Ryan, Rohay, and Sereika (1996), was concerned with the "Teleform" software for data entry and its verification.

THE USE OF COMPUTERS
FOR RESEARCH COMMUNICATION

There are two other places in the research process where computers come in handy, namely at the beginning and at the end. In reviewing the existing literature before embarking on their studies, serious researchers have available to them a number of computerized document search procedures (see, e.g., Smith, 1988). Rather than spending hours or days rummaging through various journals in the library stacks or poring over page after page in *Index Medicus,* they can type in a few key words addressed to some literature database and, before they know it, they get a list of hundreds of articles, books, unpublished reports, etc. bearing on the topic of interest. But once again, this is both a blessing and a tragedy. The same sort of speed, capacity, and accuracy that characterizes computer data analyses also is realized here, but the user is at the complete mercy of the gatherers of the database. I wish I had a nickel for every relevant article that was not picked up in a computer search but which I discovered by leafing through the key research journals. In addition, there is nothing more satisfying than a serendipitous discovery of a crucial article on a *different* topic as a byproduct of hands-on, old-fashioned digging. People who do only computer searches when they are reviewing related literature are deprived of that pleasant experience.

The end-of-process use is, of course, the employment of word processing technology in the writing of the report. Here the advantages of computerization far outweigh the disadvantages. The only real disadvantage is cost, but even that is not very high when considering some of the amazing things that word processing software can accomplish. It sounds like a simple thing, but the ability to "erase" without using up lots of paper and consuming inordinate amounts of time is absolutely priceless. In the old days, a missing comma in a dissertation could necessitate a retyping of at least one entire page. Now all we need to do is call up the document and insert the comma (the word processing program takes care of adjusting everything else), and we are all set.

I would be remiss if I did not at least mention the magnificent capabilities of computerized graphics packages such as Harvard Graphics for preparing tables and figures for manuscripts and conference presentations.

SOME SOURCES FOR
TECHNICAL MATTERS REGARDING COMPUTERS

If you would like to know more about computers and about how to write computer programs, how to use certain statistical packages, and the like, I refer you to the general article by Chang (1985) on computers and nursing research, the chapters on computers in some nursing research textbooks (e.g., Polit & Hungler, 1995), the manuals for the various statistical packages, occasional articles in the "Practical Computer" section in *Nursing Research* (two of which were cited earlier), and articles in other nursing journals on computer techniques. There also is the article by Schultz (1989) in the compendium on statistics and quantitative methods in nursing edited by Abraham, Nadzam, and Fitzpatrick (1989).

REFERENCES

Abraham, I. L., Nadzam, D. M., & Fitzpatrick, J. J. (Eds.). (1989). *Statistics and quantitative methods in nursing: Issues and strategies for research and education.* Philadelphia: W. B. Saunders.

Brennan, P. F., Moore, S. M., & Smyth, K. A. (1991). Computerlink: Electronic support for the home caregiver. *Advances in Nursing Science, 13*(4), 38-51.

Brennan, P. F., Moore, S. M., & Smyth, K. A. (1995). The effects of a special computer network on caregivers of persons with Alzheimer's disease. *Nursing Research, 44,* 166-172.

Chang, B. L. (1985). Computer use and nursing research. *Western Journal of Nursing Research, 7,* 142-144.

Davidson, L. J., Ryan, W. J., Rohay, J. M., & Sereika, S. M. (1996). Technological advances in data entry and verification: Is Teleform for you? *Nursing Research, 45,* 373-376.

Dennis, K. E. (1994). Managing questionnaire data through optical scanning technology. *Nursing Research, 43,* 376-378.

Harrison, L. L. (1989). Interfacing bioinstruments with computers for data collection in nursing research. *Research in Nursing & Health, 12,* 129-133.

Holm, R. A. (1981). Using data logging equipment. In E. E. Filsinger & R. A. Lewis (Eds.), *Assessing marriage: New behavioral approaches.* Baltimore, MD: University Park Press.

Huang, H.-Y., Wilkie, D. J., & Berry, D. L. (1996). Use of a computerized digitizer tablet to score and enter visual analogue scale data. *Nursing Research, 45,* 370-372.

Munro, B. H. (1997). *Statistics for health care research* (3rd ed.). Philadelphia: Lippincott.

Polit, D. F., & Hungler, B. P. (1995). *Nursing research: Principles and methods* (5th ed.). Philadelphia: Lippincott.

Schultz, S. (1989). The incipient paradigm shift in statistical computing. In I. L. Abraham, D. M. Nadzam, & J. J. Fitzpatrick (Eds.), *Statistics and quantitative methods in nursing: Issues and strategies for research and education* (pp. 30-36). Philadelphia: W. B. Saunders.

Smith, L. W. (1988). Microcomputer-based bibliographic searching. *Nursing Research, 37,* 125-127.

Staggers, N., & Mills, M. E. (1994). Nurse-computer interaction: Staff performance outcomes. *Nursing Research, 43,* 144-150.

White, M. A., & Wear, E. (1980). Parent-child separation: An observational methodology. *Western Journal of Nursing Research, 2,* 758-760.

White, M. A., Wear, E., & Stephenson, G. (1983). A computer-compatible method for observing falling asleep behavior of hospitalized children. *Research in Nursing & Health, 6,* 191-198.

Yarandi, H. N. (1993). Coding dummy variables and calculating the relative risk in a logistic regression. *Nursing Research, 42,* 312-314.

STUDY SUGGESTION

Choose any article in any one of your favorite nursing research journals, see what indications (if any) there are regarding the use of computers in the study reported in that article, and evaluate to what extent such use was appropriate.

PART D

SPECIALIZED
QUANTITATIVE
TECHNIQUES

This part of the book is devoted to a collection of quantitative research methods that are used in a relatively small but ever-increasing percentage of nursing studies.

Chapter 13, the first of the four chapters, concentrates on secondary analysis, in which investigators analyze data that already exist, not data that they personally have collected.

Chapter 14 treats meta-analysis (actually meta-synthesis), which can best be characterized as a statistical review of the literature.

Two approaches that often have been held in low regard, pilot studies and replication studies, are discussed together in Chapter 15. Both are absolutely crucial to the advancement of knowledge, the former being the way in which to "get the bugs out" of research plans *before* a primary study is carried out and the latter to determine *after* the primary study is carried out whether or not, or to what extent, the findings of the primary study are corroborated.

Methodological research (i.e., research on the methods used in research) is addressed in Chapter 16 along with the related matter of methodological criticism.

Secondary Analysis

Key Terms: primary analysis, secondary analysis

Many people think that all researchers collect their own data. It comes as a surprise to them to learn that there are entire disciplines (e.g., economics) in which most of the data are collected by persons other than the researchers themselves and for purposes other than the ones to which they are put by the researchers. Analyses of data that have been collected by other people for other purposes are called **secondary analyses.**

Secondary analyses are increasingly popular in nursing research. In this chapter, I describe this approach to the advancement of scientific knowledge, explain where the term comes from, discuss some of the advantages and disadvantages of secondary analysis, and give several examples of secondary analyses in the quantitative nursing research literature.

To better understand what a secondary analysis is, it is helpful to contrast that term with the term **primary analysis** (Glass, 1976). Primary analysis refers to the analysis that was carried out on the data in the original study and for the purposes for which the original study was designed.

A secondary analysis "taps into" the data collected by the people who conducted the primary analysis and operates on the data in either or both of the following ways:

1. Reanalyzes the very same data for the very same research questions, perhaps in a more sophisticated fashion

2. Uses those data, or some portions of those data, to address different research questions

SECONDARY ANALYSIS AS REANALYSIS

Reanalysis is most likely to take place when the findings of a primary analysis are controversial. Because methodological controversy is fairly rare in research in general and in nursing research in particular (perhaps rightly so given that it often has "political" overtones), secondary analyses of this type are not encountered very often in the nursing research literature. (For an unusual exception, see Johnson, Ratner, Bottorff, & Hayduk, 1993.)

SECONDARY ANALYSIS AS
AN INITIAL APPROACH TO NEW QUESTIONS

The much more common type of secondary analysis is one that asks new questions of a given database. For example, a primary analysis may have focused on the simple relationship between stress and depression at a single point in time for a combined sample of males and females; a secondary analysis of those data and additional data at a second point in time from the same data set might investigate the relationship between stress at Time 1 and depression at Time 2 for females only.

Most research projects yield more data than can be analyzed by the original investigators. In addition to studying unanalyzed variables (as illustrated by the example just given), the secondary analyst may choose to organize the data differently. The unit of analysis might be changed from the individual to some aggregate of individuals (e.g., from patient to hospital) or vice versa. (See Chapter 16 for a summary of the article by Wu, 1995, regarding one type of data analysis, hierarchical linear modeling, that uses various units of analysis). In addition, or alternatively, smaller or larger categories of data may be created that more closely relate to the current research interest or new hypothesis to be tested.

ADVANTAGES AND DISADVANTAGES OF SECONDARY ANALYSIS

The most obvious advantage of secondary analysis is the saving in time and effort by not having to collect one's own data. If the data set is the product of a well-designed study that used excellent measuring instruments, then there is the additional advantage that the quality of the data probably is better than the quality of any original data that the secondary analyst could have collected. (For these and other reasons, secondary analysis is actually preferred over primary analysis for master's theses and doctoral dissertations in some schools and colleges of nursing.)

But there are compensating disadvantages. The user of the data set is completely at the mercy of the original investigator(s), having no control whatsoever over how the data were collected; therefore, in terms of content, the data may not fit the proposed research very well. (A good scientist might "bend" the *analysis* to fit the data but *never* should bend the *question* to fit the data.)

There is more. Some data sets are very expensive to purchase. (Others, such as U.S. census data sets, have only nominal charges.) The logistics involved in transferring the data from the original investigator to the secondary analyst also can get very complicated, even with ever-increasing compatibility of output from one computer with input to another. Combining two data sets also is a prelude to some secondary analyses; that too can get tricky.

The example of U.S. census data brings up another point. The original purpose for collecting the data may not even have been a scientific one. Census data are collected every 10 years for the *political* purpose of apportioning membership in the House of Representatives. All other purposes are subordinate to that objective. It just turns out that social scientists find the information contained in census data to be a "gold mine" for answering some very interesting *scientific* questions as well.

In nursing research, secondary analyses, like pilot studies and replication studies (see Chapter 15), used to have second-class status. But the availability of large computerized data sets, combined with the realization of the tremendous cost of compiling similar data sets by individual investigators, has changed all of that. Reports of secondary analyses are finding their way into the prestige journals such as *Nursing Research* and *Research in Nursing & Health,* and at the same time they are contributing greatly to the advancement of nursing science.

SOME EXAMPLES OF
SECONDARY ANALYSES IN NURSING RESEARCH

Munro (1980) tapped into some of the data collected in the National Longitudinal Study (NLS) of the high school class of 1972 to study the problem of dropouts in nursing education. Using a sample of 363 students (129 in associate degree programs and 234 in baccalaureate programs), she tested a theoretical model of persistence. There apparently were no (or very few) problems encountered in adapting information from the data set to operationalize the constructs with which she was concerned.

In a later study, Munro (1983) used some other data collected in that same study to investigate the correlates of job satisfaction for a sample of 329 graduates of nursing programs. She was concerned with the extent to which the motivation-hygiene theory of Herzberg and his colleagues was supported by such data. Although the NLS data set was generally a very rich source of the information in which Munro was interested, she did acknowledge that the respondents had not been asked to distinguish between satisfaction and dissatisfaction (she would have done so if she had collected the data), and there were no data on the recognition motivator that is one of the elements of the theory of Herzberg and colleagues.

A third example of a secondary analysis is the work of Greenleaf (1983), to which reference already was made in Chapter 8. For her study of labor force participation of registered nurses, Greenleaf obtained data made available for public use by the National Opinion Research Center of the University of Chicago. She compared a sample of 124 registered nurses to a sample of 157 elementary school teachers and a sample of 96 "others." (All three samples consisted of females under 65 years of age.) Like Munro (1980, 1983), Greenleaf (1983) had to settle for a few minor deficiencies in the data, for example, the difficulties associated with the use of block quota sampling for some of the surveys (1972, 1973, 1974, and half of 1975 and 1976) and full probability sampling for the rest of the surveys (the other halves of 1975 and 1976 and all of 1977, 1978, and 1980). She did not say anything about what happened to 1979!

A fourth example was provided by Cohen and Loomis (1985), who studied methods of coping with stress by carrying out a linguistic analysis of responses given by 172 mental health employees to a questionnaire concerning work stress, burnout, and coping strategies. Cohen and Loomis (1985) did not discuss how the original study was designed or whether or not they experienced any difficulties with the data set; they said only that they chose a secondary analysis "because of the exploratory and preliminary nature of this work" (p. 359).

More recent examples can be found in the works of Bradley et al. (1994); Kolanowski, Hurwitz, Taylor, Evans, and Strumpf (1994); Palmer, German, and Ouslander, 1991; and Pletsch (1991). Bradley et al. (1994) explored the relationship between scores on the HOME Inventory and income, a relationship that initially had been studied as part of a randomized clinical trial. Kolanowski et al. (1994) used some data collected in a randomized clinical trial to test a model concerned with the quality of life for institutionalized elders. Palmer et al. (1991) was an analysis of risk factors for urinary incontinence of nursing home residents. Pletsch (1991) was a survey of cigarette smoking by Hispanic women.

Three other recent examples are the works of Brewer (1996); Hall, Kotch, Browne, and Rayens (1996); and Weaver, Richmond, and Narsavage (1997). Brewer's (1996) study is an example of the classic economic approach to a research problem; she analyzed some data from the National Samples of Registered Nurses for 1984 and 1988 to get some idea of the changing conditions in the supply of and demand for nurses in the labor force. Hall et al. (1996) asked some additional questions of data originally gathered by Kotch et al. (1995) to study abuse and neglect of low-income children. Weaver et al. (1997) used data previously collected by Weaver and Narsavage (1992) to test a model of the effect of various variables on functional status for patients with chronic obstructive pulmonary disease.

I had the privilege of participating in and coauthoring the reports of two secondary analyses. The first of these (Julian & Knapp, 1995) was a secondary analysis of some of the data collected in the National Survey of Families and Households (NSFH). In our article, we described the data set, pointed out some of its strengths and weaknesses, and summarized the results of an investigation of the internal consistency reliability (using Cronbach's coefficient alpha) of a set of 12 items in the survey that were excerpted from the Center for Epidemiological Studies Depression Scale (CES-D), for which we had responses from a large national subsample. This was a classic example of an analysis of data (for the CES-D) that had not been subjected to prior scrutiny in any primary analyses carried out by the original investigators.

The second of these reports (Brown, Knapp, & Radke, 1997) explored, for each of several data sets, the extent to which the readily available variables of sex, age, height, and weight can predict physiological variables such as forced expiratory volume, resting energy expenditure, and cholesterol level.

WHERE TO FIND OUT MORE
ABOUT SECONDARY ANALYSIS

The article by McArt and McDougal (1985) provides nursing researchers with an excellent introduction to secondary analysis, its advantages and disadvantages, and examples of existing data sets that are available for "dredging." The article by Lobo (1986) provides another very readable discussion of this technique. The article by Gleit and Graham (1989) describes their experiences in working with a particular data set, the Supplement on Aging tapes. The article by Ailinger, Lasus, and Choi (1997) discusses the accessing of national data sets through the latest CD-ROM technology. In addition, Sage has published two books (Kiecolt & Nathan, 1985; Stewart & Kamins, 1993) on secondary analysis in general.

REFERENCES

Ailinger, R. L., Lasus, H., & Choi, E. (1997). Using national data sets on CD-ROM to teach nursing research. *Image, 29,* 17-20.

Bradley, R. H., Mundfrom, D. J., Whiteside, L., Caldwell, B. M., Casey, P. H., Kirby, R. S., & Hansen, S. (1994). A reexamination of the association between HOME scores and income. *Nursing Research, 43,* 260-266.

Brewer, C. S. (1996). The roller coaster supply of registered nurses: Lessons from the eighties. *Research in Nursing & Health, 19,* 345-357.

Brown, J. K., Knapp, T. R., & Radke, K. J. (1997). Sex, age, height, and weight as predictors of selected physiologic outcomes. *Nursing Research, 46,* 101-104.

Cohen, M. Z., & Loomis, M. E. (1985). Linguistic analysis of questionnaire responses: Methods of coping with work stress. *Western Journal of Nursing Research, 7,* 357-366.

Glass, G. V (1976). Primary, secondary, and meta-analysis of research. *Educational Researcher, 5,* 3-8.

Gleit, C., & Graham, B. (1989). Secondary data analysis: A valuable resource. *Nursing Research, 38,* 380-381.

Greenleaf, N. P. (1983). Labor force participation among registered nurses and women in comparable occupations. *Nursing Research, 32,* 306-311.

Hall, L. A., Kotch, J. B., Browne, D. C., & Rayens, M. K. (1996). Self-esteem as a mediator of the effects of stress and social resources on depressive symptoms in postpartum mothers. *Nursing Research, 45,* 231-238.

Johnson, J. L., Ratner, P. A., Bottorff, J. L., & Hayduk, L. A. (1993). An exploration of Pender's Health Promotion Model using LISREL. *Nursing Research, 42,* 132-138.

Julian, T. W., & Knapp, T. R. (1995). The National Survey of Families and Households: A rich database for nursing research. *Research in Nursing & Health, 18,* 173-177.

Kiecolt, K. J., & Nathan, L. E. (1985). *Secondary analysis of survey data.* Beverly Hills, CA: Sage.

Kolanowski, A., Hurwitz, S., Taylor, L. A., Evans, L., & Strumpf, N. (1994). Contextual factors associated with disturbing behaviors in institutionalized elders. *Nursing Research, 43,* 73-79.

Kotch, J. B., Browne, D. C., Ringwalt, C. L., Stewart, W. P., Ruina, E., Holt, K., Lowman, B., & Jung, J. W. (1995). Risk of child abuse or neglect in a cohort of low-income children. *Child Abuse & Neglect, 19,* 1115-1130.

Lobo, M. (1986). Secondary analysis as a strategy for nursing research. In P. L. Chinn (Ed.), *Nursing research methodology* (pp. 295-304). Rockville, MD: Aspen.

McArt, E. W., & McDougal, L. W. (1985). Secondary analysis: A new approach to nursing research. *Image, 17,* 54-57.

Munro, B. H. (1980). Dropouts from nursing education: Path analysis of a national sample. *Nursing Research, 29,* 371-377.

Munro, B. H. (1983). Job satisfaction among recent graduates of schools of nursing. *Nursing Research, 32,* 350-355.

Palmer, M. H., German, P. S., & Ouslander, J. G. (1991). Risk factors for urinary incontinence one year after nursing home admission. *Research in Nursing & Health, 14,* 405-412.

Pletsch, P. K. (1991). Prevalence of smoking in Hispanic women of childbearing age. *Nursing Research, 40,* 103-106.

Stewart, D. W., & Kamins, M. A. (1993). *Secondary research: Information sources and methods* (2nd ed.). Newbury Park, CA: Sage.

Weaver, T. E., & Narsavage, G. L. (1992). Physiological and psychological variables related to functional status in chronic obstructive lung disease. *Nursing Research, 41,* 286-291.

Weaver, T. E., Richmond, T. S., & Narsavage, G. L. (1997). An explanatory model of functional status in chronic obstructive pulmonary disease. *Nursing Research, 46,* 26-31.

Wu, Y.-W. B. (1995). Hierarchical linear models: A multilevel data analysis technique. *Nursing Research, 44,* 123-126.

STUDY SUGGESTION

Look up, in a recent issue of *Nursing Research* or *Research in Nursing & Health,* an article that reports the results of a secondary analysis of existing data and answer the following questions:

a. Was this analysis a reanalysis of the same data used in the primary analysis or an analysis of data that are relevant to research questions different from those addressed in the original study?

b. What, in your opinion, was the principal advantage of the use of secondary analysis in that research report? What was the principal disadvantage? Why?

Meta-Analysis

In a **meta-analysis** (the prefix "meta" is from the Greek and means "beyond"), the principal findings of the primary analyses of several similar studies are combined (actually synthesized rather than analyzed) to produce a statistical summary of the "state of the evidence" bearing on a particular topic. This is quite different from the traditional narrative review of the literature (e.g., Lindenberg, Alexander, Gendrop, Nencioli, & Williams, 1991). The procedures for conducting meta-analyses are very complicated. Those of you who are interested in pursuing such matters are referred to Glass's (1976) article; the articles by O'Flynn (1982), Abraham and Schultz (1983), Lynn (1989), and Brown and Hedges (1994); the two monographs by Hunter and his colleagues (Hunter & Schmidt, 1990; Hunter, Schmidt, & Jackson, 1982); the textbook by Hedges and Olkin (1985); and the Sage publication by Wolf (1986).

The principal advantage of meta-analysis is the actual quantification of the literature review, giving the reader some indication of the strength of the typical finding regarding a particular phenomenon. The principal disadvantage (other than the difficulties involved in carrying out such analyses) is the determination of which studies to include in the review (Brown, 1991) and how to convert their findings to a common metric. (A post hoc version of Cohen's [1988] "effect size" is the usual choice.) Suppose, for example, that two investigators both were interested in the relationship between height and weight for adult females. One used the Smith tape measure to measure height, used the Jones scale to measure weight, and carried out a linear regression analysis. The other investigator asked the subjects to self-report their heights and weights and collapsed the data into a 2 × 2 table (height less than or equal to 64 inches and height greater than 64 inches vs. weight less than or equal to 125 pounds and weight greater than 125 pounds). "Pooling" the findings of those two studies, along with others, would be hard to do.

It also must be pointed out that having carried out a meta-analysis does not relieve the researcher of the obligation to interpret the findings of the individual studies that have been included. A meta-analysis provides no better (and no worse) context for this than does a traditional narrative review of the research literature.

SOME EXAMPLES OF META-ANALYSES

The 1995 volume of *Nursing Research* contained four interesting examples of meta-analyses. The first two were carried out by Devine and Reifschneider (1995) and Irvine and Evans (1995) and were reported in back-to-back articles in the July-August 1995 issue. The first was titled "A Meta-Analysis of the Effects of Psychoeducational Care in Adults With Hypertension" (Devine & Reifschneider, 1995). As the title implies, it was a review of 102 studies that investigated the effects of various psychological and/or educational interventions on blood pressure and related variables such as knowledge about hypertension and medication compliance. The average size of experimental effect depended largely on the actual dependent variable studied.

The second analysis was titled "Job Satisfaction and Turnover Among Nurses: Integrating Research Findings Across Studies" (Irvine & Evans, 1995). (The subtitle defines rather nicely what it is that a meta-analysis hopes to accomplish.) All of the studies reviewed by Irvine and Evans were concerned with the testing of causal models regarding job satisfaction as a mediating variable and turnover as the "ultimate" outcome variable.

The third example appeared in the very next issue and was reported by Beck (1995). Her article, titled "The Effects of Postpartum Depression on Maternal-Infant Interaction: A Meta-Analysis," summarized 19 studies on that topic. A "moderate to large" effect was found in each of them.

The fourth example followed one issue later and was titled "A Meta-Analysis of Nurse Practitioners and Nurse Midwives in Primary Care" (Brown & Grimes, 1995). It was a summary of the results of 53 studies that compared physicians to *either* nurse practitioners or nurse midwives regarding outcomes such as patient compliance and patient satisfaction.

AN EARLIER, PRACTICE-RELEVANT EXAMPLE

How should intravenous devices be irrigated? There is considerable controversy in nursing regarding the relative effectiveness of heparin flushes and saline flushes for maintaining patency, preventing phlebitis, and maximizing the duration of heparin lock placement. One way in which to help resolve such a controversy is to conduct a traditional narrative review of the empirical research literature in which reports of studies comparing one method to the other have been published. Goode et al. (1991) did not do that. They determined the average effect size of 17 studies concerned with one or more of the three dependent variables (patency, phlebitis, and duration) and found a small difference in favor of saline flushing. They also showed that the use of saline solutions is far more cost-effective. (Whether or not any changes in practice were made as a result of that study is an interesting, but separate, issue.)

For some other similar examples in nursing research, see Blegen (1993), which also was concerned with job satisfaction; Krywanio (1994); and Wilkie, Savedra, Holzemer, Tesler, and Paul (1990).

THE PRESENT STATUS OF META-ANALYSIS IN QUANTITATIVE NURSING RESEARCH

Meta-analysis now is extremely popular in nursing research. In addition to the studies already summarized here, there were eight other meta-analyses reported in the pages of *Nursing Research* from 1990 through 1996 alone, including two more by Beck (1996a, 1996b) and one by Kinney, Burfitt, Stullenbarger, Rees, and DeBolt (1996). Beck (1996c) also wrote an article *about* meta-analysis. The first issue of the 1997 volume of *Nursing Research* contained another article, by Labyak and Metzger (1997), a very brief synthesis of only nine studies that were concerned with the effects of backrubs on blood pressure and other physiological variables.

One of the recent issues of *Research in Nursing & Health* contained an article by Devine (1996) that was a report of a meta-analysis of 31 studies concerned with the psychoeducational care of adults with asthma, and an earlier article by Blue (1995) in that journal actually used a combination of meta-analysis and traditional narrative review.

This technique is even more popular in some other sciences, especially psychology. As I pointed out in Chapter 11, there is a task force in psychology that is considering the adoption of meta-analysis as the *only* method for accumulating knowledge in that discipline, completely replacing all traditional narrative reviews of related literature. I, for one, think that is going too far.

REFERENCES

Abraham, I. L., & Schultz, S. (1983). Univariate statistical models for meta-analysis. *Nursing Research, 32,* 312-315.

Beck, C. T. (1995). The effects of postpartum depression on maternal-infant interaction: A meta-analysis. *Nursing Research, 44,* 298-304.

Beck, C. T. (1996a). A meta-analysis of postpartum depression. *Nursing Research, 45,* 297-303.

Beck, C. T. (1996b). A meta-analysis of the relationship between postpartum depression and infant temperament. *Nursing Research, 45,* 225-230.

Beck, C. T. (1996c). Use of a meta-analytic database management system. *Nursing Research, 45,* 181-184.

Blegen, M. A. (1993). Nurses' job satisfaction: A meta-analysis of related variables. *Nursing Research, 42,* 36-41.

Blue, C. L. (1995). The predictive capacity of the theory of reasoned action and the theory of planned behavior in exercise research: An integrated literature review. *Research in Nursing & Health, 18,* 105-121.

Brown, S. A. (1991). Measurement of quality of primary studies for meta-analysis. *Nursing Research, 40,* 352-355.

Brown, S. A., & Grimes, D. E. (1995). A meta-analysis of nurse practitioners and nurse midwives in primary care. *Nursing Research, 44,* 332-339.

Brown, S. A., & Hedges, L. V. (1994). Predicting metabolic control in diabetes: A pilot study using meta-analysis to estimate a linear model. *Nursing Research, 43,* 362-368.

Cohen, J. (1988). *Statistical power analysis for the behavioral sciences* (2nd ed.). Hillsdale, NJ: Lawrence Erlbaum.

Devine, E. C. (1996). Meta-analysis of the effects of psychoeducational care in adults with asthma. *Research in Nursing & Health, 19,* 367-376.

Devine, E. C., & Reifschneider, E. (1995). A meta-analysis of the effects of psychoeducational care in adults with hypertension. *Nursing Research, 44,* 237-245.

Glass, G. V. (1976). Primary, secondary, and meta-analysis of research. *Educational Researcher, 5,* 3-8.

Goode, C. J., Titler, M., Rakel, B., Ones, D. Z., Kleiber, C., Small, S., & Triolo, P. K. (1991). A meta-analysis of effects of heparin flush and saline flush: Quality and cost implications. *Nursing Research, 40,* 324-330.

Hedges, L. V., & Olkin, I. (1985). *Statistical methods for meta-analysis.* San Diego, CA: Academic Press.

Hunter, J. E., & Schmidt, F. L. (1990). *Methods of meta-analysis: Correcting error and bias in research findings.* Newbury Park, CA: Sage.

Hunter, J. E., Schmidt, F. L., & Jackson, G. B. (1982). *Meta-analysis: Cumulating research findings across studies.* Beverly Hills, CA: Sage.

Irvine, D. M., & Evans, M. G. (1995). Job satisfaction and turnover among nurses: Integrating research findings across studies. *Nursing Research, 44,* 246-253.

Kinney, M. R., Burfitt, S. N., Stullenbarger, E., Rees, B., & DeBolt, M. R. (1996). Quality of life in cardiac patient research. *Nursing Research, 45,* 173-180.

Krywanio, M. L. (1994). Meta-analysis of physiological outcomes of hospital-based infant intervention programs. *Nursing Research, 43,* 133-137.

Kuhlman, G. J., Wilson, H. S., Hutchinson, S. A., & Wallhagen, M. (1991). Alzheimer's disease and family caregiving: Critical synthesis of the literature and research agenda. *Nursing Research, 40,* 331-337.

Labyak, S. E., & Metzger, B. L. (1997). The effects of effleurage backrub on the physiological components of relaxation: A meta-analysis. *Nursing Research, 46,* 59-62.

Lindenberg, C. S., Alexander, E. M., Gendrop, S. C., Nencioli, M., & Williams, D. G. (1991). A review of the literature on cocaine abuse in pregnancy. *Nursing Research, 40,* 69-75.

Lynn, M. R. (1989). Meta-analysis: Appropriate tool for the integration of nursing research? *Nursing Research, 38,* 302-305.

O'Flynn, A. (1982). Meta-analysis. *Nursing Research, 31,* 314-316.

Wilkie, D. J., Savedra, M. C., Holzemer, W. L., Tesler, M. D., & Paul, S. M. (1990). Use of the McGill Pain Questionnaire to measure pain: A meta-analysis. *Nursing Research, 39,* 36-41.

Wolf, F. M. (1986). *Meta-analysis.* Beverly Hills, CA: Sage.

STUDY SUGGESTION

Compare the meta-analysis carried out by Goode et al. (1991) in the lead article of the November-December 1991 issue of *Nursing Research* to the traditional narrative review of the literature carried out by Kuhlman, Wilson, Hutchinson, and Wallhagen (1991) in the article that immediately followed the Goode et al. (1991) article. Which approach do you prefer? Why?

CHAPTER 15

Pilot Studies and Replication Studies

Key Terms: pilot study, feasibility study, replication study, confirm, corroborate

In the preceding two chapters, I discussed secondary analyses and meta-analyses. Both of those types of studies differ from "primary" studies in which researchers do everything—phrase the research questions and/or hypotheses, design the studies, draw the samples, collect the data, and analyze the data. In this chapter, I discuss two other types of research that are not primary studies, namely pilot studies and replication studies.

In the strictest sense of the term, a **pilot study** is a miniature of a primary (main) study. Before launching the main study, the person carrying out the pilot study tries to duplicate, on a smaller scale, all the procedures that have been planned for the main study that is to follow. The purpose of a pilot study, therefore, is to try out the sampling method, test out the measuring instruments, see whether the proposed data analyses are defensible, and generally try to "get the bugs out." Preliminary studies of measuring instruments often are referred to as "pilot testing" or "pretesting." However, the term "pretesting" should not be used with respect to pilot studies; instead, it should be saved for primary experiments in which measures on the dependent variable(s) are taken both before and after certain interventions are implemented (see Chapter 5). Pilot studies also are not to be confused with **feasibility studies**; the latter are carried out on a very small number of research subjects, and their goal is the much narrower purpose of ascertaining the practicability of one or two of the proposed features of the primary study.

A **replication study**, on the other hand, is a study that is undertaken *after* a primary study has been completed to see whether the findings of an initial study are generalizable. Persons carrying out such studies typically choose one dimension with respect to which their contributions differ from the original but which are otherwise essentially the same.

For example, the hypothetical New England sex education study referred to in Chapter 3 could be replicated in Southern California on a similar sample employing the same experimental design. Or, if the New England study had been carried out for boys, then another study in that same region could be carried out for girls. Or, perhaps both dimensions could be changed; that is, the second study could concentrate on girls in Southern California. Varying more than one dimension at a time would be risky, however, because if the findings of the original study did not replicate, then the investigator would not know whether it was the sex of the subjects or the geographical location that should be "blamed."

WHY DO WE NEED PILOT STUDIES?

If any serious difficulties are encountered in carrying out a pilot study, then the researcher has the opportunity to change the procedures in the execution of the primary study to avoid those same difficulties. For example, if the data obtained in the pilot study suggested that a particular measuring instrument is invalid and/or unreliable, then the researcher might want to use another instrument—with or without another pilot study—in operationalizing the construct(s) of interest. In the absence of the pilot study, the researcher is liable to fall victim to the same measurement invalidity and/or unreliability for the main sample, at which time it would be too late to do anything about it (Prescott & Soeken, 1989).

SOME EXAMPLES OF PILOT STUDIES

There have been a number of interesting reports of pilot studies in various issues of *Nursing Research* during the past 10 years or so. They are summarized briefly here in rough chronological order.

Rice, Caldwell, Butler, and Robinson (1986) carried out a pilot study of a relaxation intervention that they had planned to implement in a later experiment investigating its effectiveness with respect to cardiac catheterization. The following year, Medoff-Cooper and Brooten (1987) reported the results of a pilot effort that involved studying the feeding cycle of a small sample of preterm infants.

The quantitative nursing research literature of the early 1990s contained reports of a few other pilot investigations. Naylor (1990) piloted a set of procedures that had been contemplated to be used in a study of discharge planning for elderly people. In that same year, Holtzclaw (1990) conducted a mini-experiment on the effect of wrappings for minimizing shivering brought on by the use of drugs.

In a very unusual combination of pilot research and methodological research (see Chapter 16), Brown and Hedges (1994) tried out the meta-analytic techniques that they were to use in a full-scale synthesis of the findings of a variety of studies concerned with the prediction of metabolic control for diabetics.

Two recent pilot efforts were reported by Lander et al. (1996) and Tulman and Fawcett (1996a, 1996b). The former study dealt with the trial of a new topical anesthetic agent, and the latter study concerned the functional status of a small sample of women with breast cancer.

Other examples include the studies carried out by Mayo, Horne, Summers, Pearson, and Helsabeck (1996); Melnyk, Alpert-Gillis, Hensel, Cable-Beiling, and Rubenstein (1997); and Miller, Hornbrook, Archbold, and Stewart (1996) that were referred to briefly in Chapter 5. Mayo et al. (1996) used a very weak pre-experimental design involving a "historical control group" in their study of heparin flush (a group of 28 patients who previously had *not* gotten the heparin flush compared to an experimental group of 23 patients who did). At the end of their article, Mayo et al. recommended that a randomized trial be carried out to test the effects of the heparin flush. Time will tell whether or not they will do so. (Some studies that are called pilot studies never are followed up by primary studies.) One very commendable feature of the Mayo et al. article, however, is that the relevant raw data for all 51 subjects were provided, and the interested reader can judge for himself or herself how comparable the two groups really were on variables other than the principal independent variable.

Melnyk et al. (1997) actually conducted a true experiment with random assignment of 30 mothers to COPE (Creating Opportunities for Parent Empowerment) or to a comparison program. (It apparently was the smallness of the sample that led the authors to refer to the study as a pilot effort.) As mentioned in Chapter 5, Miller et al. (1996) implemented a quasi-experimental design and incorporated some cost considerations in investigating the effectiveness of their home-health intervention.

WHY DO WE NEED REPLICATION STUDIES?

Although replication studies are perhaps the least highly regarded of all types of nursing research, they are among the most essential (Beck, 1994). Most researchers want to be original and design the breakthrough study rather than "just" imitating the works of others. That is a regrettable and selfish stance, however, and it reflects a seriously mistaken view of science. Because very few studies are actually based on truly random samples of the populations to which nursing researchers wish to infer, replication is the only other way in which to "buy" generalizability. Therefore, it is essential that replication studies become as automatic a part of ongoing nursing research as they are in related disciplines such as clinical medicine.

Regarding terminology, a replication study in which the findings of the initial study are supported often is said to **confirm** those findings. The proper term should be **corroborate**, not confirm, unless the replication study is itself some sort of "gold standard," which is unlikely given that both the initial study and the replication study usually are of equal status.

EXAMPLES OF REPLICATION STUDIES
IN THE NURSING RESEARCH LITERATURE

Ventura (1986) wanted to see whether the results of her previous research (Ventura, 1982) on parent coping with infant temperament would replicate. In the earlier study, she found that there were three dominant coping behavior patterns: seeking social support and self-development; maintaining family integrity; and being religious, thankful, and content. However, the first and third of these behaviors were exhibited more often by mothers than by fathers. In the later study, the coping patterns of the first study were corroborated, but the fathers in the second sample reported more responses of depression and anxiety than did the mothers.

Another example of an attempt to replicate previous research is the investigation by Fawcett, Bliss-Holtz, Haas, Leventhal, and Rubin (1986) of body image of pregnant women. The initial research by Fawcett (1978) revealed a strong similarity in spouses' patterns of change in perceived body space during and after their wives' pregnancies. That finding did not replicate; the wives in the second study showed significant changes in perceived body space between the third month of pregnancy and the second postpartal month, but there were no corresponding changes in their husbands' scores.

More recent examples include the works of Grossman, Jorda, and Farr (1994); Lucas, Atwood, and Hagaman (1993); Mahon and Yarcheski (1992); and Mishel, Padilla, Grant, and Sorenson (1991).

Grossman et al. (1994) attempted, with some success, to replicate the findings of an earlier study of blood pressure rhythms by Grossman (1990).

Lucas et al. (1993) were able to replicate the findings of previous research by Hinshaw and Atwood (1983) on turnover of nursing staff. (That research already was referred to in Chapter 11.)

Mahon and Yarcheski (1992) attempted to both replicate and extend their previous research (Mahon & Yarcheski, 1988) on loneliness in adolescents. The earlier research did not replicate; that was not surprising given that the earlier study was based on 53 boys and 59 girls between 12 and 14 years of age only, whereas the latter study examined 55 boys and 58 girls between 12 and 14 years of age *and* 31 boys and 75 girls between 15 and 17 years of age *and* 48 males and 58 females between 18 and 21 years of age.

Mishel et al. (1991) tested, with a more heterogeneous sample, the same model of uncertainty that had been tested previously by Mishel and Sorenson (1991). Some, but not all, of the relationships postulated in the model were found to replicate.

There is an entire book devoted to replication research (Neuliep, 1991). All of the examples are taken from the social sciences, but the arguments apply equally well to nursing. One of the most interesting points made in that book is the connection between replication studies and meta-analysis (see Chapter 14). As the number of replications increases, the need becomes one of summarizing the state of the science rather than of assessing whether or not an original finding can be generalized.

A POSSIBLE "SOLUTION"
TO THE REPLICATION "PROBLEM"

As I have pointed out in this chapter, replication studies are sorely needed, but hardly anyone wants to carry them out. (The examples just cited are commendable exceptions.) Every year, hundreds of master's theses are written in colleges and schools of nursing. Master's degree students often search desperately for topics—and for committees to support them. They and their advisers are painfully aware of their limitations as "full-fledged" researchers due to their minimal research training and experience. Some do narrative reviews of the research literature (frequently very good ones) on particular topics. Many more try their hands at original research, with mixed results.

It seems to me that master's theses are the ideal vehicle for replication studies. Two very important purposes would be served simultaneously. First, master's students would receive an appropriate introduction to the research process. Second, more of the necessary evidence required for the support (or lack of support) of various theories would be gathered. Doctoral students and established nursing research faculty could concentrate on the original contributions. Better yet, doctoral students and/or established faculty could work in teams with master's students to carry out both the initial works *and* the replication efforts together.

REFERENCES

Beck, C. T. (1994). Replication strategies for nursing research. *Image, 26,* 191-194.

Brown, S. A., & Hedges, L. V. (1994). Predicting metabolic control in diabetes: A pilot study using meta-analysis to estimate a linear model. *Nursing Research, 43,* 362-368.

Fawcett, J. (1978). Body image and the pregnant couple. *American Journal of Maternal Child Nursing, 3,* 227-233.

Fawcett, J., Bliss-Holtz, V. J., Haas, M. B., Leventhal, M., & Rubin, M. (1986). Spouses' body image changes during and after pregnancy: A replication and extension. *Nursing Research, 35,* 220-223.

Grossman, D. G. S. (1990). Circadian rhythms in blood pressure in school-age children of normotensive and hypertensive parents. *Nursing Research, 40,* 28-34.

Grossman, D. G. S., Jorda, M. L., & Farr, L. A. (1994). Blood pressure rhythms in early school-age children of normative and hypertensive parents: A replication study. *Nursing Research, 43,* 232-237.

Hinshaw, A. S., & Atwood, J. R. (1983). Nursing staff turnover, stress, and satisfaction: Models, measures, and management. In H. H. Werley & J. J. Fitzpatrick (Eds.), *Annual review of nursing research* (Vol. 1, pp. 133-155). New York: Springer.

Holtzclaw, B. J. (1990). Effects of extremity wraps to control drug-induced shivering: A pilot study. *Nursing Research, 39,* 280-283.

Lander, J., Nazarali, S., Hodgins, M., Friesen, E., McTavish, J., Ouellette, J., & Abel, R. (1996). Evaluation of a new topical anesthetic agent: A pilot study. *Nursing Research, 45,* 50-53.

Lucas, M. D., Atwood, J. R., & Hagaman, R. (1993). Replication and validation of Anticipated Turnover Model for urban registered nurses. *Nursing Research, 42,* 29-35.

Mahon, N. E., & Yarcheski, A. (1988). Loneliness in early adolescents: An empirical test of alternate explanations. *Nursing Research, 37,* 330-335.

Mahon, N. E., & Yarcheski, A. (1992). Alternate explanations of loneliness in adolescents: A replication and extension study. *Nursing Research, 41,* 151-156.

Mayo, D. J., Horne, M. K., III, Summers, B. L., Pearson, D. C., & Helsabeck, C. B. (1996). The effects of heparin flush on patency of the Groshong catheter. *Oncology Nursing Forum, 23,* 1401-1405.

Medoff-Cooper, B., & Brooten, D. (1987). Relation of the feeding cycle to neurobehavioral assessment in preterm infants: A pilot study. *Nursing Research, 36,* 315-317.

Melnyk, B. M., Alpert-Gillis, L. J., Hensel, P. B., Cable-Beiling, R. C., & Rubenstein, J. S. (1997). Helping mothers cope with a critically ill child: A pilot test of the COPE intervention. *Research in Nursing & Health, 20,* 3-14.

Miller, L. L., Hornbrook, M. C., Archbold, P. G., & Stewart, B. J. (1996). Development of use and cost measures in a nursing intervention for family caregivers and frail elderly patients. *Research in Nursing & Health, 19,* 273-285.

Mishel, M. H., Padilla, G., Grant, M., & Sorenson, D. S. (1991). Uncertainty in illness theory: A replication of the mediating effects of mastery and coping. *Nursing Research, 40,* 236-240.

Mishel, M. H., & Sorenson, D. S. (1991). Uncertainty in gynecological cancer: A test of the mediating functions of mastery and coping. *Nursing Research, 40,* 167-171.

Naylor, M. D. (1990). Comprehensive discharge planning for hospitalized elderly: A pilot study. *Nursing Research, 39,* 156-161.

Neuliep, J. W. (Ed.). (1991). *Replication research in the social sciences*. Newbury Park, CA: Sage.

Prescott, P. A., & Soeken, K. L. (1989). The potential uses of pilot work. *Nursing Research, 38*, 60-62.

Rice, V. H., Caldwell, M., Butler, S., & Robinson, J. (1986). Relaxation training and response to cardiac catheterization: A pilot study. *Nursing Research, 35*, 39-43.

Tulman, L., & Fawcett, J. (1996a). Biobehavioral correlates of functional status following diagnosis of breast cancer: Report of a pilot study. *Image, 28*, 181.

Tulman, L., & Fawcett, J. (1996b). Lessons learned from a pilot study of biobehavioral correlates of functional status in women with breast cancer. *Nursing Research, 45*, 356-358.

Ventura, J. N. (1982). Parent coping behaviors, parent functioning and infant temperament characteristics. *Nursing Research, 31*, 268-273.

Ventura, J. N. (1986). Parent coping: A replication. *Nursing Research, 35*, 77-80.

STUDY SUGGESTIONS

1. Look up, in the nursing research literature, an article that claims to be a pilot study and see whether or not you agree that it is a pilot study.

2. Look up another article that claims to be a replication study along with the article that reports the results of the original study. In what sense is the later study a replication of the earlier study? What dimensions have been changed? Just the sample? The instruments? The design? Is the replication study the sort of study that you think could be carried out by a master's degree student in nursing? Why or why not?

Methodological Research

Key Terms: methodological research, methodology, substance, methodological criticism

Methodological research is a very special type of research. Rather than being a way of adding to substantive knowledge, it is devoted to *studying the ways* of adding to substantive knowledge. It is research on the procedures used to carry out research, especially measuring instruments. Methodological research also includes books, journal articles, and the like that are *critiques* of research methods.

The best source for methodological research in the quantitative nursing research literature is the "Methodology Corner" section of the journal *Nursing Research*. Some issues of the journal have included several articles in that section. The November-December 1991 issue contained 7 articles that dealt with topics ranging from "Measurement of Quality of Primary

Studies for Meta-Analysis" to "Inventions and Patents." The September-October 1993 issue of that journal had 9 articles in the Methodology Corner with topics ranging from "Theoretical and Methodological Differentiation of Moderation and Mediation" to "Poster Update: Getting Their Attention." The November-December 1996 issue had 12 such articles; the first was titled "Avoiding Common Mistakes in APA Style: The Briefest of Guidelines," and the last was titled "Using the Solomon Four Design." It is obvious from the titles of these articles that the term "methodological research" is conceived rather broadly.

Several of the articles that appeared in *Nursing Research*'s Methodology Corner in the 1980s were compiled in book form by Downs (1988), who served as the editor of that journal for approximately 18 years (from 1979 through 1996).

The *Western Journal of Nursing Research* has a section called "Technical Notes" in some of its issues, in which articles similar to those in the Methodology Corner have been published. *Research in Nursing & Health* had a "Focus on Psychometrics" column for many years, which, as the name implies, was concerned with matters related to the quality of measuring instruments in nursing research. It recently has been broadened to include attention to more general quantitative matters and now bears the title "Focus on Quantitative Methods." *Research in Nursing & Health* also has a "Focus on Qualitative Methods" section.

SOME EXAMPLES OF "MAINLINE" METHODOLOGICAL RESEARCH

The typical article in a journal such as *Nursing Research* that reports the results of an investigation of the validity and/or reliability of a measuring instrument is the most common type of methodological research, and some of those already were referred to in Chapter 10. One such article appeared recently in the July-August 1995 issue of *Nursing Research*. It was titled "Development and Testing of the Barriers to Cessation Scale" (Macnee & Talsma, 1995). As its title implies, the article summarized the results of several studies that were carried out to provide some evidence regarding the validity and reliability of the Barriers to Cessation Scale, an instrument designed to assess the reasons that cigarette smokers give for being unwilling and/or unable to stop smoking. Their research addressed a method for getting at those reasons, *not* substantive matters such as whether the reasons are defensible or not, how the reasons provided relate to other variables, or the like.

Another example of methodological research that addressed measurement issues and also was concerned with "barriers" is the investigation reported by Sechrist, Walker, and Pender (1987) in an article titled "Development and Psychometric Evaluation of the Exercise Benefits Barrier Scale" that appeared in *Research in Nursing & Health* in 1987. That instrument was used to provide the data for one of the principal variables in a substantive study by Neuberger, Kasal, Smith, Hassanein, and DeViney (1994).

A third protypical example of a methodological research report is the article by Williams, Thomas, Young, Jozwiak, and Hector (1991) in which they described the development and psychometric properties of a health habits scale. A fourth example is is the work by Norwood (1996) on the Social Support Apgar. (There are several types of Apgar instruments used in quantitative nursing research, all stemming from the original infant Apgar but with the letters A, P, G, A, and R standing for different things.)

An example of a methodological contribution that was not directly concerned with instrumentation is the contribution of Wu (1995) in the Methodology Corner section of the March-April 1995 issue of *Nursing Research*. In that article, he described a technique, hierarchical linear modeling, for investigating the effects of independent variables on dependent variables for more than one unit of analysis, for example, the individual patient and an aggregate group of patients in a hospital. Unit-of-analysis problems and non-independence-of-observations problems permeate all of scientific research, and it is essential to realize that relationships found at one level do not necessarily hold at a higher or lower level.

Another example of "non-instrumentation" methodological research is the unusual study by Brown and Hedges (1994) referred to in Chapter 15. It is a combination of pilot research (they tried things out) and methodological research on meta-analysis (that is what they tried out).

OTHER EXAMPLES OF
VALIDITY AND RELIABILITY STUDIES

The January-February 1988 issue of *Nursing Research* contained three successive articles on instruments that have been developed to measure constructs of direct relevance to nursing investigations. The first article, by Miller and Powers (1988), was concerned with the measurement of hope. The next article, by Quinless and Nelson (1988), dealt with learned helplessness. The last of the three articles, by Stokes and Gordon (1988), focused on stress in the older adult. I discuss each of those articles in turn, paying particular attention to the various approaches to validity and reliability that were used in the development of the respective instruments.

Both content validity and construct validity were addressed by Miller and Powers (1988). The particular operationalization of hope that they chose was a self-report instrument called the Miller Hope Scale (MHS) in which the person indicates strength of agreement with each of 40 items by choosing one of five response categories (from *strongly disagree* to *strongly agree*). Four "judges" with substantive expertise regarding the matter of hope, along with six measurement specialists, reviewed the test and made several suggestions for modifying the items and reducing the number of items from the original 47 to the present 40. The 40-item instrument was then used in a construct validity study involving four other measures, three for convergent validity (the Psychological Well-Being Scale, the Existential Well-Being Scale, and a single-item hope self-assessment scale) and one for discriminant validity (the Hopelessness Scale). Miller and Powers found generally high positive correlations of the MHS with the other "hope-like" instruments and a –.54 correlation with the Hopelessness Scale. (They actually used the more complicated statistical technique of factor analysis.) I must point out that the Hopelessness Scale was not a good choice for discriminant validity because it is an alleged measure of the opposite of hope, not a measure of something that might be confusable with hope.

Not surprisingly, because they were dealing with a multi-item scale, Miller and Powers (1988) chose coefficient alpha as the principal determiner of the reliability of the MHS. (A sample of 522 subjects yielded a value of .93.) But to their credit, they also assessed the stability of the instrument over a 2-week period (which may have been a little long) and got a test-retest correlation of .82 based on an *N* of 308.

Quinless and Nelson (1988) also carried out a factor analysis that they claimed to provide evidence for the content, criterion-related, *and* construct validity of their Learned Helplessness Scale, a 20-item instrument using 4-point rather than 5-point item scales. (It can do nothing of the kind. Naming of the factors has some connection with content validity, but there was no "gold standard" for criterion-related validity. It was construct validity only that they studied, and just the convergent aspect at that, because they used the same Hopelessness Scale that Miller & Powers, 1988, had used and a Self-Esteem Scale [actually, lack of self-esteem] as two convergent measures.) The correlations were in the hypothesized directions but were not very strong.

For reliability assessment, Quinless and Nelson (1988) chose only coefficient alpha and obtained a coefficient of .79 for a sample of 229 participants.

Q methodology was used by Stokes and Gordon (1988) to operationalize stress. The product was the 104-item Stokes-Gordon Stress Scale. The authors claimed that content validity was guaranteed by the very way in which the scale was developed, but they reported the results of a small concurrent validity study (N was only 11) that used the Schedule of Recent Experience and the Geriatric Social Readjustment Rating Scale as external criteria.

METHODOLOGY VERSUS SUBSTANCE

I have used the terms "methodological" and "substantive" rather freely in this chapter so far. The distinction between methodology and substance is crucial. **Methodology** can be thought of as the "bones" that provide the structure for the research, and **substance** can be thought of as the "meat" of the research. Two studies could have the same bones and different meat (e.g., two experiments conducted on entirely different topics); two other studies could have the same meat and different bones (e.g., an experiment and a correlational study, both of which address the "effect" of Variable X on Variable Y).

An example of "same bones, different meat" in the nursing research literature is provided by the studies carried out by Wagner (1985) and by Zimmerman and Yeaworth (1986). They both were surveys based on simple random samples from their respective populations, but they dealt with quite different topics—smoking behavior (Wagner, 1985) and career success (Zimmerman & Yeaworth, 1986). An example of "same meat, different bones" is the pair of studies summarized by Bargagliotti (1987), one quantitative and the other qualitative, that arrived at different results regarding stress and coping. The quantitative study found that issues with management were the principal stressors, and the qualitative study found that working relationships with unit staff were the principal stressors.

A number of studies that have been "billed" as substantive contributions are really methodological investigations. The reverse situation also is fairly common (a substantive study labeled as methodological research). In the abstract preceding her article, Bradley (1983) stated, "The purpose of this study was to examine nurses' attitudes toward nursing behaviors" (p. 110). But in the body of the article, she claimed, "The major task in this investigation conducted in 1977 was to develop an instrument that would measure nurses' attitudes toward several underlying dimensions in nursing" (p. 111). It is clear from studying the article that the latter objective was the one actually pursued because almost the entire article was devoted to a factor analysis of the items and the validity and reliability of the attitude questionnaire.

One of the articles that appeared in an earlier issue of *Nursing Research* that was devoted almost exclusively to methodological research was an article on multiple triangulation by Murphy (1989b). That article was actually more substantive than methodological. Although she discussed the method of triangulation at the beginning and at the end, most of the article dealt with the findings of her research on the effects of the Mount St. Helens disaster on the bereaved survivors.

A more recent example of research that was part methodological and part substantive is the work reported by Janke (1994) regarding the Breast-Feeding Attrition Tool. In addition to providing some evidence for the validity and reliability of that instrument, the article also contained comparative data for women with breast-feeding experience versus women without prior breast-feeding experience and for women who were breast feeding versus women who were formula feeding at 8 weeks. Both of those matters are substantive, not methodological, considerations.

It is the rare study that can be both methodological and substantive. Methodological investigations should come first, in conjunction with one or more pilot studies, so that the "bugs" in the instruments, procedures for data analysis, and the like can be worked out before the major substantive studies are undertaken.

METHODOLOGICAL CRITICISM

Some of the articles in *Nursing Research*'s Methodology Corner, *Western Journal of Nursing Research*'s Technical Notes, and *Research in Nursing & Health*'s Focus on Quantitative Methods are critiques of certain research methods or the use of such methods by nursing researchers. *Nursing Research* occasionally also publishes commentaries that serve the same purpose—a very healthy purpose, in my opinion. (Methodological criticism is my specialty, and it is admittedly much easier to criticize other people's methodology than to actually carry out substantive research!)

For examples of **methodological criticism**, consider the two articles by Knapp (1990, 1993) and the article by Knapp and Brown (1995). The 1990 and 1993 articles summarized my position regarding the controversy concerning the treatment of ordinal scales as interval scales. The 1995 article took nursing researchers to task for being too tightly bound to various rules for minimum values that certain psychometric characteristics should possess.

A FINAL NOTE

In the nursing research literature, the terms "method" and "methodology" tend to be used interchangeably. For example, in describing the procedures that were followed in a substantive investigation, some authors label such a section "method," whereas others prefer the term "methodology." Strictly speaking, any word that ends in "-ology" should refer to the *study* of something, but I see no great harm done in choosing the longer term if its meaning is clear to the reader.

REFERENCES

Bargagliotti, L. A. (1987). Differences in stress and coping findings: A reflection of social realities or methodologies? *Nursing Research, 36,* 170-173.

Bradley, J. C. (1983). Nurses' attitudes toward dimensions of nursing practice. *Nursing Research, 32,* 110-114.

Brown, S. A., & Hedges, L. V. (1994). Predicting metabolic control in diabetes: A pilot study using meta-analysis to estimate a linear model. *Nursing Research, 43,* 362-368.

Downs, F. S. (1988). *Handbook of research methodology.* New York: American Journal of Nursing.

Janke, J. R. (1994). Development of the breast-feeding attrition prediction tool. *Nursing Research, 43,* 100-104.

Knapp, T. R. (1990). Treating ordinal scales as interval scales: An attempt to resolve the controversy. *Nursing Research, 39,* 121-123.

Knapp, T. R. (1993). Treating ordinal scales as ordinal scales. *Nursing Research, 42,* 184-186.

Knapp, T. R., & Brown, J. K. (1995). Ten measurement commandments that often should be broken. *Research in Nursing & Health, 18,* 465-469.

Macnee, C. L., & Talsma, A. (1995). Development and testing of the Barriers to Cessation Scale. *Nursing Research, 44,* 214-219.

Miller, J. F., & Powers, M. J. (1988). Development of an instrument to measure hope. *Nursing Research, 37,* 6-10.

Murphy, S. A. (1989b). Multiple triangulation: Applications in a program of nursing research. *Nursing Research, 38,* 294-297.

Neuberger, G. B., Kasal, S., Smith, K. V., Hassanein, R., & DeViney, S. (1994). Determinants of exercise and aerobic fitness in outpatients with arthritis. *Nursing Research, 43,* 11-17.

Norwood, S. L. (1996). The Social Support Apgar: Instrument development and testing. *Research in Nursing & Health, 19,* 143-152.

Quinless, F. W., & Nelson, M. A. M. (1988). Development of a measure of learned helplessness. *Nursing Research, 37,* 11-15.

Sechrist, K. R., Walker, S. N., & Pender, N. J. (1987). Development and psychometric evaluation of the Exercise Benefits Barrier Scale. *Research in Nursing & Health, 10,* 357-365.

Stokes, S. A., & Gordon, S. E. (1988). Development of an instrument to measure stress in the older adult. *Nursing Research, 37,* 16-19.

Wagner, T. J. (1985). Smoking behavior of nurses in western New York. *Nursing Research, 34,* 58-60.

Williams, R. L., Thomas, S. P., Young, D. O., Jozwiak, J. J., & Hector, M. A. (1991). Development of a health habits scale. *Research in Nursing & Health, 14,* 145-153.

Wu, Y.-W. B. (1995). Hierarchical linear models: A multilevel data analysis technique. *Nursing Research, 44,* 123-126.

Zimmerman, L., & Yeaworth, R. (1986). Factors influencing career success in nursing. *Research in Nursing & Health, 9,* 179-185.

STUDY SUGGESTIONS

1. In the July-August 1994 Methodology Corner of *Nursing Research,* there appeared an article by Pickett et al. (1994) titled "Use of Debriefing Techniques to Prevent Compassion Fatigue in Research Teams." Read that article. Does it belong in the Methodology Corner? Why or why not?

2. Read the article by Knapp and Brown (1995) on "commandments." Do you agree with the authors' position or do you find such rules to be necessary? Why?

MISCELLANEOUS TOPICS

The final part of this book addresses four topics that do not fit neatly anywhere else but, in my opinion, are equally as important as those that do.

Chapter 17 is concerned with the matter of "running" subjects one at a time. In much of clinical nursing research, this is exactly what happens, and it raises a number of interesting methodological issues.

How to (and whether or not to) measure change is treated in Chapter 18. Everyone is interested in measuring change, but nobody is quite sure about how to do it, and there are some sticky problems associated with change measurement that are best handled through the use of slope analysis.

Chapter 19 is devoted to the vexing problem of missing data, the bane of all quantitative nursing researchers' existence.

In Chapter 20, I try to sum up several considerations regarding the end result of any research study: the preparation of a report of the findings.

CHAPTER **17**

Running Subjects
One at a Time

Traditional data analysis tacitly assumes that research subjects have been sampled at the same time and that all are measured essentially simultaneously on the same variables. To take an ideal hypothetical example, if a random sample of 100 widgets is taken in "one fell swoop" from a conveyor belt containing a population of thousands of widgets, and if each of the 100 widgets is inspected one right after the other and determined to be defective or not defective, then the percentage of defectives in the sample is alleged to provide a reasonable estimate of the percentage of defectives in the entire population.

This matter of simultaneity of sampling and measurement turns out to be the exception rather than the rule in quantitative nursing research. Real-life research just does not work that way very often. The much more common situation is that subjects (usually people) are sampled sequentially across time and measured whenever it is convenient to do so. In a typical nursing research study, it is likely that people are enrolled in the study in dribs and drabs (often one subject at a time), measurements are taken, and the observations are entered into a database and analyzed once at the end of the study. This results in a bothersome inconsistency between how the data are gathered and how they are analyzed.

In this chapter, I discuss some of the advantages and disadvantages of "running" research subjects one at a time and suggest a more appropriate way in which to analyze the data when such is the case.

ADVANTAGES OF RUNNING
SUBJECTS ONE AT A TIME

The most obvious advantage of single-subject accumulation is that it is the way in which they usually come. Consider the common recruitment device of posting a notice indicating that subjects are needed for a certain clinical study (see, e.g., Timmerman, 1996). Potential subjects read the notice, decide whether or not they would like to participate in the study, and are deemed to satisfy or to not satisfy the inclusion and exclusion criteria. Then, at various appointed times, those who "qualify" are experimented on, interviewed, or whatever.

Another advantage is that the researcher can devote his or her individual attention to one subject at a time rather than spreading himself or herself too thin across several subjects simultaneously. Trying to manage the administration of a complicated survey instrument to, say, 100 students sitting in an auditorium is not a simple task. I know; I have had to do it more than once in my life.

A third advantage is that the measurements obtained are more likely to be independent of one another. If John's score on a questionnaire on attitudes toward abortion is obtained on Monday in Columbus, Ohio, and Mary's score on that same instrument is obtained on Friday in Rochester, New York, then one would be hard-pressed to claim that his responses influenced hers or vice versa. If they were seated next to one another in a group setting because they were husband and wife, brother and sister, or just friends, then the independence of their scores would be much more in doubt. (The only way in which to properly conduct a true experiment when subjects are run at the *same* time is to use some sort of "isolation booths" so that the subjects are not affected by other subjects in the same *or* different treatment conditions.)

DISADVANTAGES OF RUNNING
SUBJECTS ONE AT A TIME

But there are compensating disadvantage. One of these already has been mentioned, namely the tacit assumption for most analyses that the data have been gathered simultaneously rather than sequentially.

A second disadvantage is the matter of cost. It almost always is less expensive to run several subjects together than to run them separately because there is a fixed cost that must be incurred for each run as well as a variable cost associated with each subject.

A third disadvantage is the other side of the coin for the second advantage indicated in the previous section, namely that by devoting attention to one subject at a time, the researcher may consciously or unconsciously compromise his or her objectivity. Almost all quantitative nursing researchers are clinicians as well, and every effort must be made to shed the clinician's hat while carrying out the research. That is much harder to do when studying research subjects one at a time.

HOW BEST TO ANALYZE THE DATA

If the *design* is such that subjects are run one at a time (or in very small collectives), then the *analysis* should reflect that. There are two defensible ways of analyzing such data. The first and simpler way is to reconceptualize the study of N subjects as N "case studies" and to prepare N narrative reports and/or N tables or graphs that summarize the findings for the N subjects. This approach is fairly common in infant research and is the modal reporting technique in the journal *Maternal-Child Nursing*. But it also can be used for $N = 1$ experiments. (See the brief section in Chapter 5 on this topic as well as the article by Holm, 1983, the text by McLaughlin & Marascuilo, 1990, and the text by Edgington, 1995, that were cited in conjunction with such experiments.) A good example of such an approach is the research reported by Thomas (1991) regarding the monitoring of body temperature for five preterm infants. She provided individual graphs for three of the five infants as illustrations of the various patterns of biorhythms that she discovered.

A second and even more attractive way is to employ sequential analysis—either sequential hypothesis testing or sequential interval estimation. (For details regarding the former, see Brown, Porter, & Knapp, 1993.) In this approach, the researcher takes a "look" at the data after each subject (or each small group of subjects) is run and makes the decision to either stop collecting data (if a defensible inference can be made) or continue collecting data (if it cannot). To stay "honest," however, the number of looks at the data and the outcome of each look may need to be taken into account. The bad news about sequential analysis is that things can get very complicated mathematically. The good news is that the ultimate sample size required is smaller, on the average, than the sample size required for traditional power-based procedures. So far as I know, there are no real-world examples of nursing research in which sequential analysis was the method of choice, but it often should be.

ANIMAL RESEARCH

Almost nobody who carries out animal research worries enough about whether the animals are run in individual cages, in small groups, or all together in one or two environments, for example, with the experimental animals in one cage and the control animals in another. As indicated earlier and elsewhere in this book, a study should be analyzed in such a way as to reflect all of the design features. If animals are run one at a time, then their data should be summarized one at a time; if they are run in small groups, then "group" should be a factor in the analysis; and so on.

REPEATED-MEASURES
DESIGNS AND ANALYSES

Perhaps the greatest offenders of the principles alluded to in this chapter are those quantitative nursing researchers who use repeated-measures designs with time as the within-subjects factor, where the subjects are run one at a time and repeated-measures analysis of variance (ANOVA) is used to analyze the data. One of the crucial assumptions of repeated-measures ANOVA is that there is no Subject × Time interaction in the population from which the subjects have been sampled. What this means in plain English is that the patterns of scores on the dependent variable across time are essentially the same for all the subjects. If Mary's scores go up, go up again, and then go down, and if John's scores go down, go down again, and then go up, then you have a problem. There is a significance test for this assumption called Tukey's test for additivity, but hardly anybody bothers to employ it. (Assumptions are much easier to make than to test!) If Mary's pattern of scores differs from John's, then that is actually an important finding despite its being a violation of the additivity assumption for a particular type of analysis. The better strategy is to use an analysis that reflects such interesting features *and* can at the same time provide answers to the overall research questions. (See Chapter 18 for a discussion of one approach, slope analysis, that does just that.)

REFERENCES

Brown, J. K., Porter, L. A., & Knapp, T. R. (1993). The applicability of sequential analysis to nursing research. *Nursing Research, 42,* 280-282.

Edgington, E. S. (1995). *Randomization tests* (3rd ed.). New York: Marcel Dekker.

Holm, K. (1983). Single subject research. *Nursing Research, 32,* 253-255.

McLaughlin, F. E., & Marascuilo, L. A. (1990). *Advanced nursing and health care research: Quantification approaches.* Philadelphia: W. B. Saunders.

Thomas, K. A. (1991). The emergence of body temperature biorhythm in preterm infants. *Nursing Research, 40,* 98-102.

Timmerman, G. M. (1996). The art of advertising for research subjects. *Nursing Research, 45,* 339-340, 344.

STUDY SUGGESTION

Select an article in a recent issue of *Nursing Research* or *Research in Nursing & Health* in which it appears that subjects (people or animals) were run one at a time, determine whether the author(s) of the research report acknowledged that matter, and see whether or not you agree with the way in which the author(s) analyzed the data.

CHAPTER 18

The Measurement of Change

In the long chapter on measurement (Chapter 10), I intentionally avoided one of the thorniest problems in quantitative nursing research, namely the measurement of change. Nothing is more natural than having an interest in the concept of change. Does a course in sex education cause a change in attitudes toward teenage pregnancy? What is the relationship between change in income bracket and change in lifestyle? Unfortunately, nothing creates more methodological problems than the measurement of such changes. Cronbach and Furby (1970) gave a convincing argument several years ago for seriously considering giving up all attempts at intellectualizing change *and* measuring it, and some nursing researchers also have urged caution when measuring change (see, e.g., Burckhardt, Goodwin, & Prescott, 1982, and Tilden & Stewart, 1985). In this chapter, I point out some of the difficulties encountered in the measurement of change and describe one way for coping with most of them.

"SIMPLE" CHANGE

The simplest type of change is the difference between a measurement at one point in time and a measurement at a subsequent point in time. For example, consider a true experiment in which both a pretest and a posttest are employed. Subjects are randomly assigned to either an experimental group or a control group and are measured before the experiment begins and after the experiment is finished; the "treatment effect" is estimated by comparing the pre-to-post difference scores for the two groups. If the subjects in the experimental group gained more than the subjects in the control group on the average, then the experimental treatment is deemed to be better than the control treatment. (Whether or not it is statistically significantly better is a separate issue.) Everything appears to be straight-forward, right? Well, not quite.

The problem is that a difference score, here the posttest score minus the pretest score, turns out to be less reliable than either the posttest score itself or the pretest score itself. Worse yet, the degree of unreliability is greatest when the correlation between pretest score and posttest score is high. (If that correlation is not high, then it does not make much sense to subtract one from the other. It would be like mixing apples and oranges.) That obviously presents a serious dilemma. The researcher does not want to concentrate on the posttest score only because the two groups may differ, if only by chance, on the pretest, and so that should be taken into account. And this is for a true experiment. Things are even more complicated for nonrandomized treatment groups. Therefore, simple difference scores are not appropriate operationalizations of "change" unless the reliabilities of "both ends" are high and the correlation between the "ends" is low, a most unlikely eventuality. So, what should the researcher do?

THE ANALYSIS OF COVARIANCE
AND THE JOHNSON-NEYMAN TECHNIQUE

The most common alternative to an analysis of simple change scores for an experiment is the use of the analysis of covariance (ANCOVA) with type of treatment as the principal independent variable, score on the posttest as the dependent variable, and score on the pretest as the covariate. But this creates a problem. The ANCOVA has an unusually large number of assumptions that must be satisfied (see, e.g., Wu & Slakter, 1989). In addition to the traditional parametric assumptions of normality, homoscedasticity, and independence of observations, there are the assumptions of homogeneity of regression (the relationship between pretest and posttest must be the same for both treatment groups) and the independence of pretest and treatment (the score on the covariate must not be influenced by the category [experimental or control] into which a subject has been classified).

An appeal to robustness cannot be made for the homogeneity of regression assumption, but that assumption can be relaxed if the Johnson-Neyman technique is used to analyze the data rather than a strict ANCOVA (Dorsey & Soeken, 1996). The other assumption is not a problem in a true experiment (How can treatment designation affect one's score on the pretest if the pretest is taken before the experiment begins?), but in other applications of the ANCOVA it is unlikely to be satisfied. For example, if a random sample of men is compared to a random sample of women on mathematics achievement and the researcher wants to statistically control for mathematics aptitude, then the "treatment" designation (sex) could very well affect the score on the covariate (mathematics aptitude).

HOW ELSE CAN CHANGE BE
OPERATIONALIZED? (SLOPE ANALYSIS)

A few years ago, Kraemer and Thiemann (1989) proposed a technique for handling "soft data" that are gathered across time but might have "holes" due to missing observations. They suggested that change could be operationalized by calculating for each subject the **slope** of the line that best fit his or her data when the measurement on the dependent variable is plotted on the vertical axis against time as the independent variable on the horizontal axis. (See the discussion of slopes in Chapter 11.) For example, if a lung cancer patient is measured on three successive Mondays at 10 a.m. and the corresponding weights are 170, 165, and 167 pounds, then the data can be represented as follows:

X:	0	.5	1
Y:	170	165	167

The X of 0 is the first measurement, the X of 1 is the third and last measurement, and the x of .5 is halfway between.

If those data are plotted on a conventional two-dimensional graph and a regression analysis is carried out, then the slope of the line of best fit turns out to be −3.00. (The intercept is 168.83, but it is not of equal interest.) That slope can be interpreted as the average change in weight (a loss of 3 pounds) over that person's time interval. If another lung cancer patient's weight was measured on five occasions—say, Tuesday at 9 a.m., the subsequent Friday at 11 a.m., the Sunday after that at 2 p.m, the Thursday after that at 3 p.m., and the Wednesday after that at 6 p.m.—with weights of 180, 185, 180, 176, and 178 pounds, respectively, then the data for that patient are as follows:

X:	0	.201	.339	.604	1
Y:	180	185	180	176	178

The X's of 0 and 1 are again the first and last time points, and the other values of X are the proportionally intermediate values between the first time point and the last time point—a span of 369 hours.

Plotting these five data points and carrying out the associated regression analysis, a slope of −4.96 is obtained (an average loss of a little under 5 pounds).

This procedure for measuring change was endorsed by Suter, Wilson, and Naqvi (1991) and Sidani and Lynn (1993) and was used by Brown, Porter, and Knapp (1993) in their discussion of sequential hypothesis testing. I strongly recommend it for all situations in which change is of interest. It has the advantages already implied, namely that it can be used for any number of time points (including the traditional two), and the number of time points and intervals between adjacent time points can vary from subject to subject. It has the additional advantage that the only concern regarding its reliability is the number of time points; for example, a measure of change based on five time points is more reliable than a measure of change based on three time points. As I pointed out in the previous chapter, it almost always is a better choice for analyzing data collected across time than is using repeated-measures analysis of variance with all of its hard-to-satisfy assumptions. (For additional discussion of this last point, see Sidani & Lynn, 1993.)

There is one disadvantage to using a regression slope as an operationalization of change, and that is the linear aspect of this statistic. If the scatter plot forms a curvilinear, exponential, or sine-wave pattern, then the slope of the best-fitting line cannot reflect such features. But Kraemer and Thiemann (1989) also provided a convincing rebuttal to that objection to the use of slopes by appealing to a horse race analogy: It does not matter *how* a horse gets to the finish line first (by alternatively staying behind and surging ahead or by maintaining a constant lead); what matters is *that* the horse gets to the finish line first. Similarly, the average change per unit time is a good indicator of change whether the trajectory is erratic or consistent.

REFERENCES

Brown, J. K., Porter, L. A., & Knapp, T. R. (1993). The applicability of sequential analysis to nursing research. *Nursing Research, 42,* 280-282.

Burckhardt, C. S., Goodwin, L. D., & Prescott, P. A. (1982). The measurement of change in nursing research: Statistical considerations. *Nursing Research, 31,* 53-55.

Cronbach, L. J., & Furby, L. (1970). How we should measure "change"—or should we? *Psychological Bulletin, 74,* 68-80.

Dorsey, S. G., & Soeken, K. L. (1996). Use of the Johnson-Neyman technique as alternative to analysis of covariance. *Nursing Research, 45,* 363-366.

Kraemer, H. C., & Thiemann, S. (1989). A strategy to use soft data effectively in randomized controlled clinical trials. *Journal of Consulting and Clinical Psychology, 57,* 148-154.

Sidani, S., & Lynn, M. R. (1993). Examining amount and pattern of change: Comparing repeated measures ANOVA and individual regression analysis. *Nursing Research, 42,* 283-286.

Suter, W. N., Wilson, D., & Naqvi, A. (1991). Using slopes to measure directional change. *Nursing Research, 40,* 250-252.

Tilden, V. P., & Stewart, B. J. (1985). Problems in measuring reciprocity with difference scores. *Western Journal of Nursing Research, 7,* 381-385.

Wu, Y.-W. B., & Slakter, M. J. (1989). Analysis of covariance in nursing research. *Nursing Research, 38,* 306-308.

STUDY SUGGESTION

For the same article that you chose for the study suggestion at the end of Chapter 17, see whether the author(s) used the word "change" anywhere in the article.

1. If so, then how was it measured? Was that an appropriate way in which to do so? Why or why not?
2. If not, then was change of *implicit* concern even though the word "change" was not used? How was that handled?

CHAPTER 19

Strategies for Coping With Missing-Data Problems

One of the most annoying problems in quantitative nursing research (and in virtually all research) is the problem of missing data. Researchers go to great lengths to design their studies, draw their samples, administer their measuring instruments, and plan their analyses, only to find themselves victims of holes in their data. In this chapter, I attempt to define what is meant by missing data, explain how the problem of missing data comes about, discuss why it is a serious problem, and summarize what can be done about it.

DEFINITION OF MISSING DATA

Data are said to be **missing** when there is no information for one or more subjects on one or more variables in a research study. Missing data can be represented by blanks in the Subject × Variable data matrix. For example, in a questionnaire such as the original Profile of Mood States (POMS), which has 65 items, if Subject 9 fails to answer Item 37, then there would be a hole in Row 9 and Column 37 of the data matrix.

The principal consequence of missing data is that the N for each variable is not the same as the sample size N. This, in turn, has a number of serious implications for the proper interpretation of the study's findings.

Data usually are not regarded as missing if the subject was not sampled, if he or she was a nonrespondent, or if the variable is not applicable for that subject. For example, consider a survey conducted to estimate the percentage of registered nurses who are heavy cigarette smokers. A simple random sample of 1,000 registered nurses is drawn from the American Nurses Association (ANA) membership directory, a mailed questionnaire is sent out, and 500 of the 1,000 return the questionnaire. The sample size N for this study is 500. Suppose that there are three questions on the form:

1. Have you ever smoked cigarettes?
2. If so, are you currently smoking cigarettes?
3. If you are, approximately how many cigarettes do you smoke per day?

There could be a missing-data problem if any or all of the following scenarios should occur:

1. The number of responses to Question 1 is less than 500.
2. The number of responses to Question 2 is less than the number of *yes* responses to Question 1.
3. The number of responses to Question 3 is less than the number of *yes* responses to Question 2.

Although the sample size N is less than the 1,000 originally drawn and less than the total number of people listed in the ANA directory, that is *not* a missing-data problem in the usual sense of the term. If the N for Question 2 is less than 500, then that also is *not* a missing-data problem because the people who never smoked cigarettes cannot contribute to the data for that question (by design). The same is true for Question 3; the N for that question must be less than or equal to the N for Question 2.

HOW DOES IT HAPPEN?

There are several reasons for missing data. Perhaps the most common reason is unintentional lack of cooperation by one or more subjects. The most dedicated research participant occasionally can leave out part or all of a section of a self-report questionnaire by misinterpreting the directions, skipping a space on an answer sheet, or the like. A related matter is the inability of a subject to be a full participant in a study due to illness or death, moving out of town, or the like. In addition, it is possible that a large percentage of subjects may fail to answer certain questions if the instrument is very long and detailed and those questions appear on one of the last few pages.

Another reason for missing data is refusal to provide certain information because of personal objections. This is fairly common for measuring instruments that ask about one's income, religious beliefs, or sexual behavior.

A third reason, and one that rarely, if ever, is mentioned in the research literature, is malicious intent. It is conceivable that certain subjects (e.g., undergraduate sophomores) might intentionally fail to provide certain data because they think that the study is silly or a waste of time, and so they do all that they can to "louse things up." (They also can louse things up, for example, by providing outlier data points in claiming that they smoke 10 packs of cigarettes a day!)

The fourth reason has to do with omissions that are attributable to equipment failure, clerical problems in the gathering of the data, and problems in the entry of the data. Many of these are matters over which the principal investigators have little or no control. Examples of such situations are when (a) a slide projector that is used to provide visual stimuli burns out a bulb, (b) an interviewer neglects to ask a particular question of a given subject, and (c) a research assistant entering the data for a given subject leaves blank a bit of information that the subject did provide and the original questionnaires have inadvertently been destroyed.

WHY IS THE MISSING-DATA PROBLEM SERIOUS?

If the only analyses that are to be carried out are simple frequency distributions for each variable separately, then missing data do not pose a problem and may actually be quite informative. The fact that, say, 100 out of 500 people do not respond to a particular question may be interesting in its own right. But whenever that is not the case, which is almost always, missing data produce very bothersome consequences. Some of these are as follows.

1. Missing data drive readers up the wall. To have data in this table based on an N of 437 and data in that table based on an N of 392, for example, makes a research report very hard to read, understand, and evaluate. Matters become even worse if the N differs from variable to variable in the *same* table. (For an interesting example of the latter, see Tables 3 and 4 in Gulick, 1991.)

2. When there is no information for a variable, then it may cause data to be missing on other computed variables to which the variable contributes; therefore, a snowball effect is created. If the variable is a questionnaire item, then a subject for whom the datum is missing would not have a subscale score for the subscale to which an item belongs. Whenever all subscale scores are needed to compute a total score, it too would be missing.

3. It is difficult, if not impossible, to compare a statistic based on one sample to a statistic based on a subset of that sample. For example, if a mean at Time 1 is based on 200 people and the corresponding mean at Time 2 is based on 175 of those people, then how can one properly determine whether or not there has been a change from Time 1 to Time 2? If the 25 people who dropped out of the study between Time 1 and Time 2 had not done so, then the results might have been very different.

4. Certain analyses cannot be carried out when there are missing data; for example, regression analyses, which permeate much of nursing research, require full data for every subject. It is possible to display in a correlation matrix Pearson correlation coefficients between variables where the N's for the correlations differ from one cell to the other, but if anything is done further with such a matrix (e.g., any type of multivariate

Table 19.1   Hypothetical Data That Yield Inconsistent Correlations

Subject	W	X	Y
A	1	1	
B	2	2	
C	3	3	
D	4	4	
E	5	5	
F	1		1
G	2		2
H	3		3
I	4		4
J	5		5
K		1	5
L		2	4
M		3	3
N		4	2
O		5	1

NOTE: $r_{wx} = +1$, $r_{wy} = +1$, $r_{xy} = -1$.

analysis), then the results could be meaningless. Certain correlation coefficients are inconsistent with one another and never can hold for full data but could be produced when data are missing. (See Table 19.1 for a set of hypothetical data, with several holes, that produces such a pattern.)

5. Related to the previous problem, yet a separate concern, is the possibility that a missing-data code (9, 99, 999, etc. are the most popular codes) will be taken for real data. If, say, all the actual data range from 0 to 50 and there are a few 99's thrown in by mistake, then the results can be badly distorted.

WHAT CAN BE DONE ABOUT IT?

There exists a vast methodological literature regarding what to do about missing data, ranging from journal articles and sections in textbooks concerning relatively simple but very helpful suggestions (see, e.g., Brick & Kalton, 1996; Cohen & Cohen, 1983; Marascuilo & Levin, 1983; Tabachnick & Fidell, 1996) to an entire book on the subject (Little & Rubin, 1987).

The important thing to realize is that *all* recommendations for handling missing data are at best only that—recommendations. There is no panacea.

Strategies for coping with the problem of missing data are of five types: (a) prevent it, (b) delete additional data, (c) impute estimates for the missing data, (d) work around it, and (e) study it. I consider them in that order.

PREVENTION

The best way in which to handle missing data is to prevent the data from being missing in the first place. In many instances, the researcher can prevent missing data through anticipation of data collection problems and by good communication with data collectors. An especially critical time for missing-data prevention is when a study is just beginning. The principal investigators and research assistants should realize the need for taking the extra time to try to ensure that all the items on a questionnaire are answered by all subjects.

Another strategy to prevent missing data is to clearly address issues of subject burden with respect to both type and duration of burden. Some subjects may not be able to complete all the instruments originally planned to be administered at a given time point, and a change from a written questionnaire to a verbal interview may be called for, especially for older people (Gilmer, Cleary, Morris, Buckwalter, & Andrews, 1993). By breaking up the data collection into two or more sessions and by making the measurement procedures more conducive to subject preference, the problem of missing data may be prevented.

Another prevention strategy is to carefully examine the research instruments. Any instrument that requires subjects to answer questions on the back of a page may yield missing data unless the instruction to turn over the page is explicitly given. Researchers also should make sure that the response format of instruments is clear. Subjects may need more explicit directions about the format and/or to be given the opportunity to practice with sample items.

Prevention of missing data when questionnaires are returned in the mail can be challenging. It frequently happens that subjects return questionnaires with items omitted. The forms should be promptly inspected on receipt; if items have been omitted, then the matter should be addressed immediately. A problem arises when it is unclear whether the person intended to omit the item or whether it was an oversight. One way in which to handle this is to photocopy the instrument that was returned and mail the copy back to the subject with the omitted items highlighted. A letter could accompany the instrument saying something like, "These items were missing; if you intended not to answer the items, please disregard this letter, but if they were omitted because of oversight, please answer the highlighted questions and return the questionnaire in the envelope provided." This strategy is, of course, not available if subjects do not provide their names and addresses and when anonymity is promised because there would be no way in which to trace the sender.

A problem encountered in longitudinal studies, particularly studies of patients following a cardiac event such as angioplasty or bypass surgery, is that subjects may think that the instrument does not pertain to them because they are doing well clinically. Subjects should be informed when they enter a study about the importance of answering all the questionnaires at all time points, whether or not there have been any changes in their illnesses, and this message should be reinforced periodically throughout the study.

For more physiologically based research, equipment failures can be a major source of missing data, as already pointed out. Regular maintenance of equipment should be a part of every study. For tape recorders, it may be advisable to have extra tapes attached to the recorders or to mark on the recorders when the batteries were last changed. Protocols should be established so that data collectors know what to do if a piece of equipment fails.

To many data collectors, a questionnaire is a questionnaire and they may not have the information or knowledge to decide which of the instruments are most important. It is prudent to discuss contingency plans with data collectors for situations in which they suspect the data collection period is going to be shortened. Research assistants may use up too much time collecting demographic data that could be obtained elsewhere or at a later time and not have time collecting data on key variables that never will be available again, for example, baseline data prior to a major event such as surgery.

DELETION

If prevention strategies fail, then the researcher must decide how the problem of missing data will be handled. One option that frequently is chosen in research is, believe it or not, the deletion of additional data! One or more of the following options may be appropriate.

1. If a subject has any missing data whatsoever, then delete the subject from all analyses. This is the so-called **listwise deletion** option that is available in many computer packages. It is the most conservative approach to the handling of missing data, but at the same time it is the most wasteful. In the extreme, if every subject has just one piece of missing data and this approach were to be adopted, then there would be nothing left to analyze. In longitudinal studies, the problem is compounded because each additional time point increases the risk that the subject will be thrown out of the analysis because of missing data. For example, if total mood disruption as measured by the monopolar POMS is examined over three time periods, then there would be 195 opportunities (65 items for three time points) for a subject to be deleted. The loss of subjects, particularly in a small sample, means a loss of statistical power to detect relationships or differences and increases the chance of a Type II error (accepting a false null hypothesis).

2. If a subject has missing data for one or more variables, then delete the subject from all correlational analyses that pertain to that (those) variable(s) but retain the subject for all other analyses. This is the so-called **pairwise deletion** option that also is available in many computer packages. It is fine for merely displaying certain data but is inappropriate for more complicated analyses. Prior to running any data analyses using various computer packages, it is essential to determine what the "default" is regarding missing data. For some, it is listwise; for others, it is pairwise; and for still others, there is no default (the user must specify what is to be done regarding missing data, what missing value codes are to be used, etc.).

3. If a particular analysis requires a balanced design (e.g., a certain type of factorial analysis of variance) and the deletion of one or more subjects for whatever reason produces an unbalanced design, then randomly discard other subjects to regain the balance. This is a surprisingly frequent strategy but is not necessary (because you can run the analysis as a regression that does not require proportional cell frequencies) and could result in the fractionalization of samples that are often small to begin with. It probably goes without saying, but missing-data problems are more serious for small samples than for large samples.

4. If there is a great deal of data missing for a particular variable, then delete that variable. This is a radical strategy because there must have been

an important reason for including the variable in the study initially, and this option should be considered only as a last resort.

IMPUTATION

Imputation is a process in which the subject is given a value for an observation that is missing. The goal of the process is to impute a value that has the highest likelihood of reflecting what the actual value would have been. Imputation has been given greater attention in the literature than has deletion, principally because it is felt to be a shame to delete any data that researchers have devoted so much time and energy to collecting in the first place. Some of the recommendations are as follows.

1. If a subject has a missing datum for a variable, then impute the mean for the group (or impute the median if the variable [e.g., income] is badly skewed). This is far and away the most common imputation strategy, but it also is one of the worst. Why?

   a. The frequency distribution for the actual data might be such that the mean is not one of the scale points and/or it does not make any sense. This would be the case, for example, if the distribution were bimodal with, say, half of the scores equal to 0 and the other half equal to 10. How is a score of 5 to be interpreted?

   b. If the data have been collected in an experiment, then the treatment effect could be artificially inflated. This is because the resulting within-group variance is smaller than it otherwise would be for full data (more observations right at the mean), producing a smaller "error term" for assessing the statistical significance of the effect. This is bad science. "Stacking the deck" *against* a hypothesized treatment effect is one thing, but at least it is conservative; stacking the deck *in favor* of a hypothesized effect is something else.

   c. For a nonexperimental study, the investigator may choose to impute an item mean for the responding subjects to subjects having missing data for that item. The disadvantage of this method is that it restricts the range of scores for the item and may actually artificially lower the reliability for a subscale, thereby reducing the likelihood that strong relationships will be demonstrated between variables.

2. If a subject has a missing datum for an item on a test, then impute his or her mean on the other items. This is a variation of the previous recommendation. Its principal disadvantage is the artificial *increase* in the internal consistency reliability of the measuring instrument. Cronbach's alpha, for example, increases as the interitem correlations increase (all other things being equal), and imputing item responses that are similar to the responses for other items will raise such correlations and make the instrument look more reliable than it actually is.

3. Use common sense to impute missing data. For example, if a subject does not indicate what sex he or she is but claims to be suffering from prostate cancer, then the subject is male. (This does not work as well for a subject with breast cancer because there are a few males who do contract that disease.) This approach is a favorite strategy used by the U.S. Bureau of the Census. That organization also occasionally stretches the definition of "common sense." If a census form indicates that in a particular household there is a 35-year-old male, a 31-year-old female, and a 7-year-old child but there is no indication as to marital or parental status, the bureau might very well assume that the two adults are married to one another and that the child is their child and impute such data. This imputation strategy is less likely to have been used in the 1990 census than in, say, the 1890 census due to the various changes in lifestyles in the intervening years.

4. Use regression analysis for the subjects for whom full data are available to "predict" what the missing data might have been on the "criterion" variable for the subjects for whom only partial data are available. Although this sounds rather bizarre, it is one of the more defensible strategies provided that the associated R^2 is very high and that the subjects for whom data are missing can be assumed to be representative of the same population for which the analysis sample is representative. For example, if functional status were the variable for which data were missing and it were highly correlated with age, sex, and number of comorbidities, then the researcher could derive a regression equation predicting functional status from those three variables. The equation would then be used to estimate a subject's functional status value by plugging the individual subject's age, sex, and number of comorbidities into the regression equation. Regression-based imputation can be a logistical nightmare, however, if several regression equations are needed to impute different pieces of missing data.

5. Use one or more of the recommendations in Little and Rubin's (1987) text, for example, the estimation maximation algorithm. These are not for the methodologically faint of heart and may not be worth the effort.

If imputation is used in conjunction with any inferential statistical analysis, then it is essential that the appropriate number of degrees of freedom be taken into account. For one-way analysis of variance, for example, 1 degree of freedom must be subtracted from both the "within" and "total" degrees of freedom for each value that is imputed.

WORKING AROUND THE PROBLEM

There is an old saying that goes something like this: "If your life consists of one lemon after another, then take advantage of it and make lemonade." There are some situations in which missing data are a "blessing" and the researcher can capitalize on that information. An example already was given earlier regarding a simple frequency distribution for which "missing" is one of the categories for a variable. Two other examples now follow.

If a researcher is interested in monitoring change across time for a particular variable such as weight, then it often happens that some measurements are not available for some subjects for some time points. That could be very disappointing, but if "change" is operationalized as the slope of the best-fitting line for each subject (see Brown, Porter, & Knapp, 1993; Kraemer & Thiemann, 1989; Sidani & Lynn, 1993; Suter, Wilson, & Naqvi, 1991; and Chapter 18 of this text), then it does not present a serious problem for data analysis other than the fact that some slopes are based on three observations, others on five observations, and so on. Furthermore, the time points can vary from subject to subject, which makes such a strategy particularly attractive for clinical studies in which subjects are "run" one at a time (see Chapter 17) with different numbers of time points and different intervals between time points.

Another example is the situation in which matched pairs of subjects are desired (e.g., women and their husbands) but data are missing for one of the members of various pairs (e.g., pairs for whom there are wife data but no husband data, other pairs for whom there are husband data but no wife data). For an example of the former situation, see Northouse, Jeffs, Cracchiolo-Caraway, Lampman, & Dorris, 1995, and Northouse, Laten, & Reddy, 1995. This ordinarily would present a serious dilemma for data analysis because the two samples (one sample of wives and the other sample of husbands) are partially dependent and partially independent, so that a dependent sample t test or z test and an independent sample t test or z test both would be indefensible. Fortunately, there exist "hybrid" tests (Lin & Stivers, 1974; Thomson, 1995) that use all the available data, necessitating neither deletion nor imputation.

STUDYING THE MISSING-DATA PROBLEM

In their text, Cohen and Cohen (1983) described a method for creating "missingness" variables, that is, dichotomous variables for which the dummy variable codes of 1 and 0 can be used to indicate whether or not the datum for a subject is missing for a particular variable. The relationship between missingness and the variables of original concern can be explored with potentially interesting results. For example, it might be of some relevance to discover that there was a strong correlation between self-esteem and whether or not income was reported.

The usual best case, however, is when the missingness is independent of any of the other variables in the study; that is, whether the data are present or absent for a particular variable has no relationship with the other variables. Returning to the example of elders who were physically unable to answer a written questionnaire on their own, suppose that the study had been examining the impact of symptomatology and use of coping strategies on emotional well-being in the elderly and the researchers had *not* chosen to administer the coping questionnaire by interview format. If fatigue was the reason why the elders could not complete the coping inventory, then the fact that the data were missing would be dependent on symptomatology, another one of the independent variables. Because the data would be missing for that subset of the sample, the coping behaviors of subjects with poorer functional status would not be reflected in the analysis. Therefore, it is a good idea to examine the data matrix carefully to assess whether there is dependence between the pattern of missing data and variables in the study. If it appears that the absence of data is related to some variable, then it would be important for the researcher to explore this further. One technique for assessing independence or dependence would be to compare subjects with complete data to subjects with missing data on demographic variables or key study variables. If there were differences between subjects with missing data and those with full data, then it would suggest that there is dependence in the data. When this occurs, the lack of independence should be reported in the research report and the impact of nonindependence should be addressed in the study limitations.

TWO REAL-DATA EXAMPLES
TO ILLUSTRATE SOME OF THESE STRATEGIES

There were two recent articles in *Nursing Research* that are exemplary for their handling of missing data. Both of these articles were reports of factor analyses, and both were cited previously in Chapter 10. In the first article, by Wineman, Durand, and McCulloch (1994), the authors included a section describing what missing data problems they encountered and how each was addressed. The following are examples:

1. Subjects were dropped if they had missing data for more than 10% of the items missing for any scale.
2. Items were dropped if more than 5% of the subjects did not respond to those items.
3. Regression-based imputation was used for subjects who had small amounts of missing data.

Nice.

The second article was by Fawcett and Knauth (1996). Their "rules," formulated before they collected the data, were similar to those of Wineman et al. (1994), namely:

1. Subjects were dropped if they had more than 10% missing data.
2. An item was dropped if more than 5% of the subjects had missing data for that item. (It turned out that none of the items had to be dropped.)
3. The item mode was imputed for all other subjects who had any missing data.

Equally nice.

SO WHERE DOES THIS LEAVE US?

The problem of missing data is a bear. The best way in which to deal with it is, of course, by prevention (i.e., to not have any), but that is very hard to accomplish in research on human subjects. When it comes to a choice of delete versus impute, delete is more defensible if the amount of missing data is small and the sample is large. If imputation is necessary, then some sort of mixture of common sense and regression prediction is likely to be the most fruitful. Working around the missing-data problem and studying it are perhaps the most attractive strategies because they use all available data.

REFERENCES

Brick, J. M., & Kalton, G. (1996). Handling missing data in survey research. *Statistical Methods in Medical Research, 5,* 215-238.

Brown, J. K., Porter, L. A., & Knapp, T. R. (1993). The applicability of sequential analysis to nursing research. *Nursing Research, 42,* 280-282.

Cohen, J., & Cohen, P. (1983). *Applied multiple regression/correlation analysis for the behavioral sciences* (2nd ed.). Hillsdale, NJ: Lawrence Erlbaum.

Fawcett, J., & Knauth, D. (1996). The factor structure of the Perception of Birth Scale. *Nursing Research, 45,* 83-86.

Gilmer, J. S., Cleary, T. A., Morris, W. W., Buckwalter, K. C., & Andrews, P. (1993). Instrument format issues in assessing the elderly: The Iowa Self-Assessment Inventory. *Nursing Research, 42,* 297-299.

Gulick, E. E. (1991). Reliability and validity of the Work Assessment Scale for persons with multiple sclerosis. *Nursing Research, 40,* 107-112.

Kraemer, H. C., & Thiemann, S. (1989). A strategy to use soft data effectively in randomized controlled clinical trials. *Journal of Consulting and Clinical Psychology, 57,* 148-154.

Lin, P.-E., & Stivers, L. E. (1974). On differences of means with incomplete data. *Biometrika, 61,* 325-334.

Little, R. J. A., & Rubin, D. B. (1987). *Statistical analysis with missing data.* New York: John Wiley.

Marascuilo, L. A., & Levin, J. R. (1983). *Multivariate statistics in the social sciences.* Pacific Grove, CA: Brooks/Cole.

Northouse, L. L., Jeffs, M., Cracchiolo-Caraway, A., Lampman, L., & Dorris, G. (1995). Emotional distress reported by women and husbands prior to a breast biopsy. *Nursing Research, 44,* 196-201.

Northouse, L. L., Laten, D., & Reddy, P. (1995). Adjustment of women and their husbands to recurrent breast cancer. *Research in Nursing & Health, 18,* 515-524.

Sidani, S., & Lynn, M. R. (1993). Examining amount and pattern of change: Comparing repeated measures ANOVA and individual regression analysis. *Nursing Research, 42,* 283-286.

Suter, W. N., Wilson, D., & Naqvi, A. (1991). Using slopes to measure directional change. *Nursing Research, 40,* 250-252.

Tabachnick, B. G., & Fidell, L. S. (1996). *Using multivariate statistics* (3rd ed.). New York: HarperCollins.

Thomson, P. C. (1995). A hybrid paired and unpaired analysis for the comparison of proportions. *Statistics in Medicine, 14,* 1463-1470.

Wineman, N. M., Durand, E. J., & McCulloch, B. J. (1994). Examination of the factor structure of the Ways of Coping Questionnaire with clinical populations. *Nursing Research, 43,* 268-273.

STUDY SUGGESTION

Look up a quantitative nursing research article in which a missing-data problem occurred and write a brief critique of how the researcher(s) coped with that problem.

CHAPTER 20

The Dissemination of Research Results

It is one thing to properly design a study and to carry out a primary analysis, secondary analysis, or meta-analysis of the data. It is quite another thing to report the results of such a study in a way that is as concise and as straightforward as possible. I end this book by discussing some important considerations in the communication of quantitative nursing research findings.

THE MANUSCRIPT

Whether the basis of the communication is to be a book, a journal article, a dissertation, or a conference presentation, the starting point usually is the preparation of a manuscript that contains the information that the researcher(s) would like to convey to the audience. This involves a few rather obvious but crucial decisions. A brief discussion of, and some personal recommendations regarding, some of those decisions now follows.

WHO SHOULD WRITE IT?

The principal investigator(s) should, of course, be the principal author(s), but consultants to the research team for various aspects of the study also may be asked to write up those portions of the report for which they have special expertise.

WHO SHOULD BE
LISTED AS THE AUTHOR(S)?

This sounds like the same question, but it is not. For many clinical studies, it is fairly common practice for the researcher(s) to include as authors, out of professional courtesy, nurses and/or physicians who provided access to the research subjects but who played no part (and often have little or no interest) in the preparation of the manuscript. This can result in a paper that has as many as 10 or more authors (see, e.g., Dodd et al., 1996). Nativio (1993) and Flanagin (1993) recently provided several guidelines regarding the matter of authorship and the more delicate matter of fraudulent publication.

IN WHAT ORDER
SHOULD THE NAMES BE LISTED?

You would not believe the time and effort that go into such a decision. Should the first author be the person who has contributed the most to the study itself, the second author the person who contributed the next most, and so on? (Researchers' academic promotions, or nonpromotions, often depend on the order of their "authorships.") Or, should the authors be listed in alphabetical order in a humble show of collegiality? For a "spoof" of this and associated aspects of scientific publication, see my article in *Nurse Educator* (Knapp, 1997).

HOW LONG SHOULD THE MANUSCRIPT BE?

Doctoral dissertations are generally very long and notoriously redundant. Journal articles, on the other hand, are much shorter, with the actual length often controlled by the editorial policy of the journal—much to the dismay of individual authors. The author of a book generally has much more freedom regarding its length. All research reports, however, should be long enough to provide the essential information but not so long that they get repetitive and/or boring. Some of us are naturally verbose; others of us (including me) write too tightly. In research dissemination as in most other aspects of life, it is well to try to strike a happy medium.

HOW MANY MANUSCRIPTS
SHOULD BE GENERATED FROM ONE STUDY?

This would seem to be a simple problem to resolve—one study, one manuscript, right? Unfortunately, it is not that simple, and this issue has been the subject of a great deal of recent controversy. (See Aaronson, 1994; Blancett, Flanagin, & Young, 1995; Yarbro, 1995; and the letters to the editor of *Image* that were written in response to the Blancett et al., 1995, article.) Those who argue for multiple manuscripts per study claim that (a) the findings of a study, particularly a very large study, cannot be summarized properly in a single manuscript; (b) different manuscripts are necessary for different audiences (e.g., nurse researchers and nurse clinicians); and/or (c) some studies have methodological implications as well as substantive ones. Those on the opposite side of this issue argue that multiple manuscripts pertaining to the same study often are annoyingly redundant with one another, are not properly cited with respect to one another, and take up valuable book and journal space that could be better devoted to the reports of other studies. My personal opinion is that too much precious journal space is taken up by reports of findings of only slightly different aspects of a single study.

WHAT TYPE OF FORMAT
SHOULD BE EMPLOYED?

One of the most common formats used by (actually required by) many nursing research journals is the American Psychological Association (APA) style (APA, 1994). Some of its features can be a bit tricky; a recent article by Damrosch and Damrosch (1996) provided some very helpful guidelines.

SHOULD THERE BE ANY
TABLES AND/OR FIGURES?

Most quantitative nursing research studies are based on some conceptual framework and generate lots of data that need to be summarized in some useful fashion. Figures are appropriate for models that are to be tested and for displaying some of the data. Tables are generally more useful for summarizing most of the data, and there are likely to be more tables than figures. (It occasionally is difficult to determine the difference between a figure and a table.) The 1994 APA manual contains some excellent suggestions for figures and tables, and as indicated earlier in this book, I have tried to provide some guidelines for reporting the results of regression analyses (Knapp, 1994a); Jacobsen and Meininger (1986) discussed the same sorts of problems in the reporting of the findings of randomized clinical trials.

TO WHAT OUTLET(S) SHOULD
THE MANUSCRIPT(S) BE SUBMITTED
FOR FURTHER CONSIDERATION?

The typical publication outlet for nursing research manuscripts is one or more of the several dozen "refereed" (peer-reviewed) nursing research journals, among which a few (*Nursing Research, Research in Nursing & Health,* and a couple others) are regarded as the most prestigious. There are several other non-nursing journals that publish nursing research reports; findings of the Nurses' Health Study, for example, never have been published in a nursing research journal. I recommmend the consideration of more than one outlet because the probability is fairly high that the manuscript will get rejected by your first choice, particularly if it is one of the more highly regarded journals (Knapp, 1994b; Swanson & McCloskey, 1982; Swanson, McCloskey, & Bodensteiner, 1991). It is unethical, however, to submit a manuscript to two or more journals simultaneously. Careful consideration also should be given to the intended audience. You should not choose a more prestigious general-purpose journal over a less prestigious specialty journal if the readers of the latter journal are those you are trying to reach.

REFERENCES

Aaronson, L. S. (1994). Milking data or meeting commitments: How many papers from one study? *Nursing Research, 43,* 60-62.

American Psychological Association. (1994). *Publication manual of the American Psychological Association* (4th ed.). Washington, DC: Author.

Blancett, S. S., Flanagin, A., & Young, R. K. (1995). Duplicate publication in the nursing literature. *Image, 27,* 51-56.

Damrosch, S., & Damrosch, G. D. (1996). Avoiding common mistakes in APA style: The briefest of guidelines. *Nursing Research, 45,* 331-333.

Dodd, M. J., Larson, P. J., Dibble, S. L., Miaskowski, C., Greenspan, D., MacPhail, L., Hauck, W. W., Paul, S. M., Ignoffo, R., & Shiba, G. (1996). Randomized clinical trial of chlorhexidine versus placebo for prevention of oral mucositis in patients receiving chemotherapy. *Oncology Nursing Forum, 23,* 921-927.

Flanagin, A. (1993). Fraudulent publication. *Image, 25,* 359.

Jacobsen, B. S., & Meininger, J. C. (1986). Randomized experiments in nursing: The quality of reporting. *Nursing Research, 35,* 379-382.

Knapp, T. R. (1994a). Regression analyses: What to report. *Nursing Research, 43,* 187-189.

Knapp, T. R. (1994b). Supply (of journal space) and demand (by assistant professors). *Image, 26,* 247.

Knapp, T. R. (1997). The prestige value of books and journal articles. *Nurse Educator, 22,* 10-11.

Nativio, D. G. (1993). Authorship. *Image, 25,* 358.

Swanson, E. A., & McCloskey, J. C. (1982). The manuscript review process. *Image, 14,* 72-76.

Swanson, E. A., McCloskey, J. C., & Bodensteiner, A. (1991). Publishing opportunities for nurses: A comparison of 92 U.S. journals. *Image, 23,* 33-38.

Yarbro, C. H. (1995). Duplicate publication: Guidelines for nurse authors and editors. *Image, 27,* 57.

STUDY SUGGESTION

Read (or at least skim) all of the articles by Mercer, Ferketich, and their colleagues that were cited in Chapter 8. Do you think that there were too many articles generated from that study? Not enough? Why or why not?

References

Aaronson, L. S. (1989). A cautionary note on the use of stepwise regression. *Nursing Research, 38,* 309-311. (11)

Aaronson, L. S. (1994). Milking data or meeting commitments: How many papers from one study? *Nursing Research, 43,* 60-62. (20)

Aaronson, L. S., Frey, M. A., & Boyd, C. J. (1988). Structural equation models and nursing research: Part II. *Nursing Research, 37,* 315-317. (11)

Aaronson, L. S., & Kingry, M. J. (1988). A mixed method approach for using cross-sectional data for longitudinal inferences. *Nursing Research, 37,* 187-189. (8)

Abraham, I. L. (1994). Does suboptimal measurement reliability constrain the explained variance in regression? *Western Journal of Nursing Research, 16,* 447-452. (10)

Abraham, I. L., Nadzam, D. M., & Fitzpatrick, J. J. (Eds.). (1989). *Statistics and quantitative methods in nursing: Issues and strategies for research and education.* Philadelphia: W. B. Saunders. (12)

Abraham, I. L., & Schultz, S. (1983). Univariate statistical models for meta-analysis. *Nursing Research, 32,* 312-315. (14)

Achenbach, T. M. (1978). *Research in developmental psychology.* New York: Free Press. (8)

Acorn, S., Ratner, P. A., & Crawford, M. (1997). Decentralization as a determinant of autonomy, job satisfaction, and organizational commitment among nurse managers. *Nursing Research, 46,* 52-58. (11)

Ailinger, R. L., Lasus, H., & Choi, E. (1997). Using national data sets on CD-ROM to teach nursing research. *Image, 29,* 17-20. (13)

Allan, J. D., Mayo, K., & Michel, Y. (1993). Body size values of white and black women. *Research in Nursing & Health, 16,* 323-333. (8)

Allen, J. K. (1996). Coronary risk factor modification in women after coronary artery bypass surgery. *Nursing Research, 45,* 260-265. (5)

AUTHOR'S NOTE: The numbers in parentheses at the end of each entry refer to the chapter in which the reference is cited.

Alt-White, A. C. (1995). Obtaining "informed" consent from the elderly. *Western Journal of Nursing Research, 17,* 700-705. (4)

American Nurses Association. (1980). *Nursing: A social policy statement.* Kansas City, MO: Author. (1)

American Nurses Association. (1985). *Human rights guidelines for nurses in clinical and other research.* Kansas City, MO: Author. (4)

American Nurses Association. (1995). *Nursing's social policy statement.* Washington, DC: Author. (1)

American Psychological Association. (1994). *Publication manual of the American Psychological Association* (4th ed.). Washington, DC: Author. (20)

American Statistical Association. (varying dates). *What is a survey?* Washington, DC: Author. (6)

Anderson, K. L. (1995). The effect of chronic obstructive pulmonary disease on quality of life. *Research in Nursing & Health, 18,* 547-556. (11)

Armstrong, G. D. (1981). The intraclass correlation as a measure of interrater reliability of subjective judgments. *Nursing Research, 30,* 314-320. (10)

Baillie, V., Norbeck, J. S., & Barnes, L. A. (1988). Stress, social support, and psychological distress of family caregivers of the elderly. *Nursing Research, 37,* 217-222. (7)

Baker, N. C., Bidwell-Cerone, S., Gaze, N., & Knapp, T. R. (1984). The effect of type of thermometer and length of time inserted on oral temperature measurements of afebrile subjects. *Nursing Research, 33,* 109-111. (5, 11)

Ballard, S., & McNamara, R. (1983). Quantifying nursing needs in home health care. *Nursing Research, 32,* 236-241. (6)

Bargagliotti, L. A. (1987). Differences in stress and coping findings: A reflection of social realities or methodologies? *Nursing Research, 36,* 170-173. (16)

Barhyte, D. Y., Redman, B. K., & Neill, K. M. (1990). Population or sample: Design decision. *Nursing Research, 39,* 309-310. (11)

Baron, R. M., & Kenny, D. A. (1986). The moderator-mediator variable distinction in social psychological research: Conceptual, strategic, and statistical considerations. *Journal of Personality and Social Psychology, 51,* 1173-1182. (3)

Beck, C. T. (1994). Replication strategies for nursing research. *Image, 26,* 191-194. (15)

Beck, C. T. (1995). The effects of postpartum depression on maternal-infant interaction: A meta-analysis. *Nursing Research, 44,* 298-304. (2, 14)

Beck, C. T. (1996a). A meta-analysis of postpartum depression. *Nursing Research, 45,* 297-303. (14)

Beck, C. T. (1996b). A meta-analysis of the relationship between postpartum depression and infant temperament. *Nursing Research, 45,* 225-230. (14)

Beck, C. T. (1996c). Use of a meta-analytic database management system. *Nursing Research, 45,* 181-184. (14)

Beck, S. L. (1989). The crossover design in clinical nursing research. *Nursing Research, 38,* 291-293. (5)

Berk, R. A. (1990). Importance of expert judgment in content-related validity evidence. *Western Journal of Nursing Research, 12,* 659-671. (10)

Berry, D. L., Dodd, M. J., Hinds, P. S., & Ferrell, B. R. (1996). Informed consent: Process and clinical issues. *Oncology Nursing Forum, 23,* 507-512. (4)

Berry, J. K., Vitalo, C. A., Larson, J. L., Patel, M., & Kim, M. J. (1996). Respiratory muscle strength in older adults. *Nursing Research, 45,* 154-159. (8)

Beyer, J. E., & Aradine, C. R. (1986). Content validity of an instrument to measure young children's perceptions of the intensity of their pain. *Journal of Pediatric Nursing, 1,* 386-395. (10)

Beyer, J. E., & Aradine, C. R. (1988). Convergent and discriminant validity of a self-report measure of pain intensity for children. *Children's Health Care, 16,* 274-282. (10)

Beyer, J. E., & Knapp, T. R. (1986). Methodological issues in the measurement of children's pain. *Children's Health Care, 14,* 233-241. (10)

Blair, C. E. (1995). Combining behavior management and mutual goal setting to reduce physical dependency in nursing home residents. *Nursing Research, 44,* 160-165. (5)

Blancett, S. S., Flanagin, A., & Young, R. K. (1995). Duplicate publication in the nursing literature. *Image, 27,* 51-56. (20)

Blegen, M. A. (1993). Nurses' job satisfaction: A meta-analysis of related variables. *Nursing Research, 42,* 36-41. (14)

Blegen, M. A., Goode, C., Johnson, M., Mass, M., Chen, L., & Moorhead, S. (1993). Preferences for decision-making autonomy. *Image, 25,* 339-344. (9)

Blue, C. L. (1995). The predictive capacity of the theory of reasoned action and the theory of planned behavior in exercise research: An integrated literature review. *Research in Nursing & Health, 18,* 105-121. (14)

Bottorff, J. L., Johnson, J. L., Ratner, P. A., & Hayduk, L. A. (1996). The effects of cognitive-perceptual factors on health promotion behavior maintenance. *Nursing Research, 45,* 30-36. (11)

Bowles, C. (1986). Measure of attitude toward menopause using the semantic differential model. *Nursing Research, 35,* 81-86. (10)

Boyd, C. J., Frey, M. A., & Aaronson, L. S. (1988). Structural equation models and nursing research: Part I. *Nursing Research, 37,* 249-252. (11)

Bradley, J. C. (1983). Nurses' attitudes toward dimensions of nursing practice. *Nursing Research, 32,* 110-114. (16)

Bradley, R. H., Mundfrom, D. J., Whiteside, L., Caldwell, B. M., Casey, P. H., Kirby, R. S., & Hansen, S. (1994). A reexamination of the association between HOME scores and income. *Nursing Research, 43,* 260-266. (13)

Brandt, P. A. (1984). Stress-buffering effects of social support on maternal discipline. *Nursing Research, 33,* 229-234. (7)

Brennan, P. F., Moore, S. M., & Smyth, K. A. (1991). Computerlink: Electronic support for the home caregiver. *Advances in Nursing Science, 13*(4), 38-51. (12)

Brennan, P. F., Moore, S. M., & Smyth, K. A. (1995). The effects of a special computer network on caregivers of persons with Alzheimer's disease. *Nursing Research, 44,* 166-172. (2, 12)

Brewer, C. S. (1996). The roller coaster supply of registered nurses: Lessons from the eighties. *Research in Nursing & Health, 19,* 345-357. (13)

Brick, J. M., & Kalton, G. (1996). Handling missing data in survey research. *Statistical Methods in Medical Research, 5,* 215-238. (19)

Brink, C. A., Sampselle, C. M., & Wells, T. J. (1989). A digital test for pelvic muscle strength in older women with urinary incontinence. *Nursing Research, 38,* 196-199. (1)

Brown, J. K. (1996). Role clarification: Rights and responsibilities of oncology nurses. In R. McCorkle, M. Grant, M. Frank-Stromborg, & S. Baird (Eds.), *Cancer nursing: A comprehensive textbook* (2nd ed., pp. 1376-1387). Philadelphia: W. B. Saunders. (4)

Brown, J. K., Knapp, T. R., & Radke, K. J. (1997). Sex, age, height, and weight as predictors of selected physiologic outcomes. *Nursing Research, 46,* 101-104. (11, 13)

Brown, J. K., Porter, L. A., & Knapp, T. R. (1993). The applicability of sequential analysis to nursing research. *Nursing Research, 42,* 280-282. (17, 18, 19)

Brown, L. P., Arnold, L., Allison, D., Klein, M. E., & Jacobsen, B. (1993). Incidence and pattern of jaundice in healthy breast-fed infants during the first month of life. *Nursing Research, 42,* 106-110. (11)

Brown, S. A. (1991). Measurement of quality of primary studies for meta-analysis. *Nursing Research, 40,* 352-355. (14)

Brown, S. A., & Grimes, D. E. (1995). A meta-analysis of nurse practitioners and nurse midwives in primary care. *Nursing Research, 44,* 332-339. (14)

Brown, S. A., & Hedges, L. V. (1994). Predicting metabolic control in diabetes: A pilot study using meta-analysis to estimate a linear model. *Nursing Research, 43,* 362-368. (14, 15, 16)

Burckhardt, C. S., Goodwin, L. D., & Prescott, P. A. (1982). The measurement of change in nursing research: Statistical considerations. *Nursing Research, 31,* 53-55. (18)

Burman, M. E. (1995). Health diaries in nursing research and practice. *Image, 27,* 147-152. (10)

Butz, A. M., & Alexander, C. (1991). Use of health diaries with children. *Nursing Research, 40,* 59-61. (10)

Byra-Cook, C. J., Dracup, K. A., & Lazik, A. J. (1990). Direct and indirect blood pressure in critical care patients. *Nursing Research, 39,* 285-288. (10)

Byrne, T. J., & Edeani, D. (1984). Knowledge of medical terminology among hospital patients. *Nursing Research, 33,* 178-181. (10)

Campbell, D. T., & Fiske, D. W. (1959). Convergent and discriminant validation by the multitrait-multimethod matrix. *Psychological Bulletin, 56,* 81-105. (10)

Campbell, D. T., & Stanley, J. C. (1966). *Experimental and quasi-experimental designs for research.* Chicago: Rand McNally. (3, 5)

Campos, R. G. (1994). Rocking and pacifiers: Two comforting interventions for heelstick pain. *Research in Nursing & Health, 17,* 321-331. (5)

Carruth, A. K., Tate, U. S., Moffett, B. S., & Hill, K. (1997). Reciprocity, emotional well-being, and family functioning as determinants of family satisfaction in caregivers of elderly patients. *Nursing Research, 46,* 93-100. (11)

Carson, M. A. (1996). The impact of a relaxation technique on the lipid profile. *Nursing Research, 45,* 271-276. (2)

Chalmers, T., Smith, H., Blackburn, B., Silverman, B., Schroeder, B., Reitman, D., & Ambroz, A. (1981). A method for assessing the quality of a randomized control trial. *Controlled Clinical Trials, 2,* 31-49. (5)

Chang, B. L. (1985). Computer use and nursing research. *Western Journal of Nursing Research, 7,* 142-144. (12)

Christen, W. G., Glynn, R. J., Manson, J. E., Ajani, U. A., & Buring, J. E. (1996). A prospective study of cigarette smoking and risk of age-related macular degeneration in men. *Journal of the American Medical Association, 276,* 1147-1151. (6)

Christman, N. J., & Johnson, J. E. (1981). The importance of research in nursing. In Y. M. Williamson (Ed.), *Research methodology and its application in nursing* (pp. 3-24). New York: John Wiley. (1)

Cline, M. E., Herman, J., Shaw, E. R., & Morton, R. D. (1992). Standardization of the visual analogue scale. *Nursing Research, 41,* 378-380. (10)

Cobb, E. B. (1985). Planning research studies: An alternative to power analysis. *Nursing Research, 34,* 386-388. (9)

Coffman, S., Levitt, M. J., & Brown, L. (1994). Effects of clarification of support expectations in prenatal couples. *Nursing Research, 43,* 111-116. (11)

Cohen, J. (1960). A coefficient of agreement for nominal scales. *Educational and Psychological Measurement, 20,* 37-46. (10)

Cohen, J. (1988). *Statistical power analysis for the behavioral sciences* (2nd ed.). Hillsdale, NJ: Lawrence Erlbaum. (9, 11, 14)

Cohen, J., & Cohen, P. (1983). *Applied multiple regression/correlation analysis for the behavioral sciences* (2nd ed.). Hillsdale, NJ: Lawrence Erlbaum. (19)

Cohen, M. Z., & Loomis, M. E. (1985). Linguistic analysis of questionnaire responses: Methods of coping with work stress. *Western Journal of Nursing Research, 7,* 357-366. (13)

Colditz, G. A., Bonita, R., Stampfer, M. J., Willett, W. C., Rosner, B., Speizer, F. E., & Hennekens, C. H. (1988). Cigarette smoking and risk of stroke in middle-aged women. *New England Journal of Medicine, 318,* 937-941. (6)

Colditz, G. A., Hankinson, S. E., Hunter, D. J., Willett, W. C., Manson, J. E., Stampfer, M. J., Hennekens, C. H., Rosner, B., & Speizer, F. E. (1995). The use of estrogens and progestins and the risk of breast cancer in postmenopausal women. *New England Journal of Medicine, 332,* 1589-1593. (6)

Colditz, G. A., Martin, P., Stampfer, M. J., Willett, W. C., Sampson, L., Rosner, B., Hennekens, C. H., & Speizer, F. E. (1986). Validation of questionnaire information on risk factors and disease outcomes in a prospective cohort of women. *American Journal of Epidemiology, 123,* 894-900. (6)

Colditz, G. A., Stampfer, M. J., Willett, W. C., Stason, W. B., Rosner, B., Hennekens, C. H., & Speizer, F. E. (1987). Reproducibility and validity of self-reported menopausal status in a prospective cohort study. *American Journal of Epidemiology, 126,* 319-325. (6)

Colditz, G. A., Willett, W. C., Hunter, D. J., Stampfer, M. J., Manson, J. E., Hennekens, C. H., Rosner, B. A., & Speizer, F. E. (1993). Family history, age, and risk of breast cancer. *Journal of the American Medical Association, 270,* 338-343. (6)

Colditz, G. A., Willett, W. C., Stampfer, M. J., Rosner, B., Speizer, F. E., & Hennekens, C. H. (1987). A prospective study of age at menarche, parity, age at first birth, and coronary heart disease in women. *American Journal of Epidemiology, 126,* 861-870. (6)

Colditz, G. A., Willett, W. C., Stampfer, M. J., Sampson, M. J., Rosner, B., Hennekens, C. H., & Speizer, F. E. (1987). The influence of age, relative weight, smoking, and alcohol intake on the reproducibility of a dietary questionnaire. *International Journal of Epidemiology, 16,* 392-398. (6)

Conlon, M., & Anderson, G. (1990). Three methods of random assignment: Comparison of balance achieved on potentially confounding variables. *Nursing Research, 39,* 376-379. (3)

Cook, T. D., & Campbell, D. T. (1979). *Quasi-experimentation.* Chicago: Rand McNally. (5)

Cowan, M. E., & Murphy, S. A. (1985). Identification of postdisaster bereavement risk predictors. *Nursing Research, 34,* 71-75. (8)

Coward, D. D. (1996). Self-transcendence and correlates in a healthy population. *Nursing Research, 45,* 116-121. (7)

Cox, C. L., Sullivan, J. A., & Roghmann, K. J. (1984). A conceptual explanation of risk-reduction behavior and intervention development. *Nursing Research, 33,* 168-173. (10)

Cronbach, L. J. (1951). Coefficient alpha and the internal structure of tests. *Psychometrika, 16,* 297-334. (10)

Cronbach, L. J., & Furby, L. (1970). How we should measure "change"—or should we? *Psychological Bulletin, 74,* 68-80. (18)

Curtin, L., & Flaherty, M. J. (1982). *Nursing ethics: Theories and pragmatics.* Bowie, MD: Brady. (4)

Damrosch, S., & Damrosch, G. D. (1996). Avoiding common mistakes in APA style: The briefest of guidelines. *Nursing Research, 45,* 331-333. (20)

Darlington, R. B. (1990). *Regression and linear models.* New York: McGraw-Hill. (11)

Davidson, L. J., Ryan, W. J., Rohay, J. M., & Sereika, S. M. (1996). Technological advances in data entry and verification: Is Teleform for you? *Nursing Research, 45,* 373-376. (12)

Deiriggi, P. M. (1990). Effects of waterbed flotation on indicators of energy expenditure in preterm infants. *Nursing Research, 39,* 140-146. (1)

DeKeyser, F. G., & Pugh, L. C. (1990). Assessment of the reliability and validity of biochemical measures. *Nursing Research, 39,* 314-316. (10)

DeMaio-Esteves, M. (1990). Mediators of daily stress and perceived health status in adolescent girls. *Nursing Research, 39,* 360-364. (3, 11)

Dennis, K. E. (1986). Q methodology: Relevance and application to nursing research. *Advances in Nursing Science, 8*(3), 6-17. (10)

Dennis, K. E. (1987). Dimensions of client control. *Nursing Research, 36,* 151-156. (10)

Dennis, K. E. (1988). Q methodology: New perspectives on estimating reliability and validity. In O. L. Strickland & C. F. Waltz (Eds.), *Measurement of nursing outcomes,* Vol. 2: *Measuring nursing performance* (pp. 409-419). New York: Springer. (10)

Dennis, K. E. (1990). Patients' control and the information imperative: Clarification and confirmation. *Nursing Research, 39,* 162-166. (10)

Dennis, K. E. (1994). Managing questionnaire data through optical scanning technology. *Nursing Research, 43,* 376-378. (12)

Department of Health and Human Services. (1981, January 26). *Final regulations amending basic HHS policy for the protection of human research subjects.* Washington, DC: Author. (4)

Devine, E. C. (1996). Meta-analysis of the effects of psychoeducational care in adults with asthma. *Research in Nursing & Health, 19,* 367-376. (14)

Devine, E. C., & Reifschneider, E. (1995). A meta-analysis of the effects of psychoeducational care in adults with hypertension. *Nursing Research, 44,* 237-245. (14)

DiIorio, C., Hennessy, M., & Manteuffel, B. (1996). Epilepsy self-management: A test of a theoretical model. *Nursing Research, 45,* 211-217. (11)

Dodd, M. J., Larson, P. J., Dibble, S. L., Miaskowski, C., Greenspan, D., MacPhail, L., Hauck, W. W., Paul, S. M., Ignoffo, R., & Shiba, G. (1996). Randomized clinical trial of chlorhexidine versus placebo for prevention of oral mucositis in patients receiving chemotherapy. *Oncology Nursing Forum, 23,* 921-927. (5, 20)

Donnelley, S., & Nolan, K. (Eds.). (1990). Animals, science, and ethics. A special supplement to the *Hastings Center Report, 20*(3), 1-32. (4)

Dorsey, S. G., & Soeken, K. L. (1996). Use of the Johnson-Neyman technique as alternative to analysis of covariance. *Nursing Research, 45,* 363-366. (5, 18)

Douglas, S., Briones, J., & Chronister, C. (1994). The incidence of reporting consent rates in nursing research articles. *Image, 26,* 35-40. (4)

Douglas, S., Daly, B. J., Rudy, E. B., Sereika, S. M., Menzel, L., Song, R., Dyer, M. A., & Mintenegor, H. D. (1996). Survival experience of chronically critically ill patients. *Nursing Research, 45,* 73-77. (5)

Downs, F. S. (1988). *Handbook of research methodology.* New York: American Journal of Nursing. (16)

Duffy, M. E., Rossow, R., & Hernandez, M. (1996). Correlates of health-promotion activities in employed Mexican American women. *Nursing Research, 45,* 18-24. (2)

Edgington, E. S. (1995). *Randomization tests* (3rd ed.). New York: Marcel Dekker. (3, 5, 17)

Elifson, K. W., Runyon, R. P., & Haber, A. (1982). *Fundamentals of social statistics.* Reading, MA: Addison-Wesley. (11)

England, M., & Roberts, B. L. (1996). Theoretical and psychometric analysis of caregiver strain. *Research in Nursing & Health, 19,* 499-510. (10)

Engstrom, J. L. (1988). Assessment of the reliability of physical measures. *Research in Nursing & Health, 11,* 383-389. (10)

Engstrom, J. L., & Chen, E. H. (1984). Prediction of birthweight by the use of extrauterine measurements during labor. *Research in Nursing & Health, 7,* 314-323. (10)

Fawcett, J. (1978). Body image and the pregnant couple. *American Journal of Maternal Child Nursing, 3,* 227-233. (15)

Fawcett, J., Bliss-Holtz, V. J., Haas, M. B., Leventhal, M., & Rubin, M. (1986). Spouses' body image changes during and after pregnancy: A replication and extension. *Nursing Research, 35,* 220-223. (15)

Fawcett, J., & Knauth, D. (1996). The factor structure of the Perception of Birth Scale. *Nursing Research, 45,* 83-86. (10, 19)

Feinstein, A. R. (1985). *Clinical epidemiology.* Philadelphia: W. B. Saunders. (8)

Ferketich, S. L., & Mercer, R. T. (1994). Predictors of paternal role competence by risk status. *Nursing Research, 43,* 80-85. (8)

Ferketich, S. L., & Mercer, R. T. (1995a). Paternal-infant attachment of experienced and inexperienced fathers during infancy. *Nursing Research, 44,* 31-37. (2, 8)

Ferketich, S. L., & Mercer, R. T. (1995b). Predictors of role competence for experienced and inexperienced fathers. *Nursing Research, 44,* 89-95. (8)

Ferketich, S. L., & Verran, J. (1986). Exploratory data analysis: Introduction. *Western Journal of Nursing Research, 8,* 464-466. (11)

Ferketich, S. L., & Verran, J. (1994). An overview of data transformation. *Research in Nursing & Health, 17,* 393-396. (11)

Fetter, M. S., Feetham, S. L., D'Apolito, K., Chaze, B. A., Fink, A., Frink, B. B., Hougart, M. K., & Rushton, C. H. (1989). Randomized clinical trials: Issues for researchers. *Nursing Research, 38,* 117-120. (5)

Fieler, V. K., Wlasowicz, G. S., Mitchell, M. L., Jones, L. S., & Johnson, J. E. (1996). Information preferences of patients undergoing radiation therapy. *Oncology Nursing Forum, 23,* 1603-1608. (1)

Flanagin, A. (1993). Fraudulent publication. *Image, 25,* 359. (20)

Flaskerud, J. H. (1988). Is the Likert scale format culturally biased? *Nursing Research, 37,* 185-186. (10)

Floyd, J. A. (1993). Systematic sampling: Theory and clinical methods. *Nursing Research, 42,* 290-293. (9)

Flynn, L. (1997). The health practices of homeless women: A causal model. *Nursing Research, 46,* 72-77. (11)

Fox, R. N. (1982). Agreement corrected for chance. *Research in Nursing & Health, 5,* 45-46. (10)

Franck, L. S. (1986). A new method to quantitatively describe pain behavior in infants. *Nursing Research, 35,* 28-31. (10)

Friedman, L. M., Furberg, C. D., & DeMets, D. L. (1996). *Fundamentals of clinical trials* (3rd ed.). St. Louis, MO: Mosby. (5)

Froman, R. D., & Owen, S. V. (1997). Further validation of the AIDS Attitude Scale. *Research in Nursing & Health, 20,* 161-167. (10)

Ganong, L. H., & Coleman, M. (1992). The effect of clients' family structure on nursing students' cognitive schemas and verbal behavior. *Research in Nursing & Health, 15,* 139-146. (5)

Gilliss, C. L., & Kulkin, I. L. (1991). Monitoring nursing interventions and data collection in a randomized clinical trial. *Western Journal of Nursing Research, 13,* 416-422. (5)

Gilmer, J. S., Cleary, T. A., Morris, W. W., Buckwalter, K. C., & Andrews, P. (1993). Instrument format issues in assessing the elderly: The Iowa Self-Assessment Inventory. *Nursing Research, 42,* 297-299. (19)

Giovannetti, P. (1981). Sampling techniques. In Y. M. Williamson (Ed.), *Research methodology and its application to nursing* (pp. 169-190). New York: John Wiley. (9)

Given, B. A., Keilman, L. J., Collins, C., & Given, C. W. (1990). Strategies to minimize attrition in longitudinal studies. *Nursing Research, 39,* 184-186. (8)

Glass, G. V (1976). Primary, secondary, and meta-analysis of research. *Educational Researcher, 5,* 3-8. (13, 14)

Gleit, C., & Graham, B. (1989). Secondary data analysis: A valuable resource. *Nursing Research, 38,* 380-381. (13)

Golding, J. M. (1996). Sexual assault history and limitations in physical functioning in two general population samples. *Research in Nursing & Health, 19,* 33-44. (9)

Goldsmith, J. W. (1981). Methodological considerations in using videotape to establish rater reliability. *Nursing Research, 30,* 124-127. (10)

Good, M. (1995). A comparison of the effects of jaw relaxation and music on postoperative pain. *Nursing Research, 44,* 52-57. (5)

Goode, C. J., Titler, M., Rakel, B., Ones, D. Z., Kleiber, C., Small, S., & Triolo, P. K. (1991). A meta-analysis of effects of heparin flush and saline flush: Quality and cost implications. *Nursing Research, 40,* 324-330. (14)

Goodwin, L. D., & Prescott, P. A. (1981). Issues and approaches to estimating interrater reliability in nursing research. *Research in Nursing & Health, 4,* 323-337. (10)

Greenleaf, N. P. (1983). Labor force participation among registered nurses and women in comparable occupations. *Nursing Research, 32,* 306-311. (8, 13)

Gross, D. (1991). Issues related to validity of videotaped observational data. *Western Journal of Nursing Research, 13,* 658-663. (10)

Gross, D., Conrad, B., Fogg, L., Willis, L., & Garvey, C. (1993). What does the NCATS measure? *Nursing Research, 42,* 260-265. (10)

Gross, D., Conrad, B., Fogg, L., Willis, L., & Garvey, C. (1995). A longitudinal study of maternal depression and preschool children's mental health. *Nursing Research, 44,* 96-101. (2, 7)

Grossman, D. G. S. (1990). Circadian rhythms in blood pressure in school-age children of normotensive and hypertensive parents. *Nursing Research, 40,* 28-34. (15)

Grossman, D. G. S., Jorda, M. L., & Farr, L. A. (1994). Blood pressure rhythms in early school-age children of normative and hypertensive parents: A replication study. *Nursing Research, 43,* 232-237. (15)

Gulick, E. E. (1987). Parsimony and model confirmation of the ADL Self-Care Scale for multiple sclerosis persons. *Nursing Research, 36,* 278-283. (9)

Gulick, E. E. (1991). Reliability and validity of the Work Assessment Scale for persons with multiple sclerosis. *Nursing Research, 40,* 107-112. (10, 19)

Gunderson, L. P., Stone, K. S., & Hamlin, R. L. (1991). Endotracheal suctioning-induced heart rate alterations. *Nursing Research, 40,* 139-143. (4)

Gurklis, J. A., & Menke, E. M. (1988). Identification of stressors and use of coping methods in chronic hemodialysis patients. *Nursing Research, 37,* 236-239, 248. (9)

Gurney, C. A., Mueller, C. W., & Price, J. L. (1997). Job satisfaction and organizational attachment of nurses holding doctoral degrees. *Nursing Research, 46,* 163-171. (11)

Guttman, L. (1941). The quantification of a class of attributes: A theory and method for scale construction. In P. Horst (Ed.), *The prediction of personal adjustment* (pp. 319-348). New York: Social Science Research Council. (10)

Hall, L. A., & Farel, A. M. (1988). Maternal stresses and depressive symptoms: Correlates of behavior problems in young children. *Nursing Research, 37,* 156-161. (11)

Hall, L. A., Kotch, J. B., Browne, D. C., & Rayens, M. K. (1996). Self-esteem as a mediator of the effects of stress and social resources on depressive symptoms in postpartum mothers. *Nursing Research, 45,* 231-238. (11, 13)

Hanna, K. (1993). Effect of nurse-client transaction on female adolescents' oral contraceptive adherence. *Image, 25,* 285-290. (5)

Hanson, M. J. S. (1997). The theory of planned behavior applied to cigarette smoking in African-American, Puerto Rican, and non-Hispanic white teenage families. *Nursing Research, 46,* 155-162. (11)

Harris, R. J. (1985). *A primer of multivariate statistics* (2nd ed.). New York: Academic Press. (11)

Harrison, L. L. (1989). Interfacing bioinstruments with computers for data collection in nursing research. *Research in Nursing & Health, 12,* 129-133. (12)

Hash, V., Donlea, J., & Walljasper, D. (1985). The telephone survey: A procedure for assessing educational needs of nurses. *Nursing Research, 34,* 126-128. (6)

Hedges, L. V., & Olkin, I. (1985). *Statistical methods for meta-analysis.* San Diego, CA: Academic Press. (14)

Heidenreich, T., & Giuffre, M. (1990). Postoperative temperature measurement. *Nursing Research, 39,* 153-155. (10)

Heidenreich, T., Giuffre, M., & Doorley, J. (1992). Temperature and temperature measurement after induced hypothermia. *Nursing Research, 41,* 296-300. (10)

Heise, D. R. (1969). Separating reliability and stability in test-retest correlation. *American Sociological Review, 34,* 93-101. (10)

Hennekens, C. H., & Buring, J. E. (1987). *Epidemiology in medicine.* Boston: Little, Brown. (5, 6, 8)

Hennekens, C. H., Buring, J. E., Manson, J. E., Stampfer, M., Rosner, B., Cook, N. R., Belanger, C., LaMotte, F., Gaziano, J. M., Ridker, P. M., Willett, W., & Peto, R. (1996). Lack of evidence of long-term supplementation with beta carotene on the incidence of malignant neoplasms and cardiovascular disease. *New England Journal of Medicine, 334,* 1145-1149. (5, 6)

Hennekens, C. H., Rosner, B., Belanger, C., Speizer, F. E., Bain, C. J., & Peto, R. (1979). Use of permanent hair dyes and cancer among registered nurses. *Lancet, 79*(2), 1390-1393. (6)

Hennekens, C. H., et al. for members of the Steering Committee of the Physicians' Health Study Research Group. (1989). Final report on the aspirin component of the ongoing Physicians' Health Study. *New England Journal of Medicine, 321,* 129-135. (5, 6)

Hill, M. N., & Schron, E. B. (1992). Opportunities for nurse researchers in clinical trials. *Nursing Research, 41,* 114-116. (5)

Hinds, P. S., & Young, K. J. (1987). A triangulation of methods and paradigms to study nurse-given wellness care. *Nursing Research, 36,* 195-198. (10)

Hinshaw, A. S., & Atwood, J. R. (1983). Nursing staff turnover, stress, and satisfaction: Models, measures, and management. In H. H. Werley & J. J. Fitzpatrick (Eds.), *Annual review of nursing research* (Vol. 1, pp. 133-155). New York: Springer. (15)

Holland, P. W. (1986). Statistics and causal inference. *Journal of the American Statistical Association, 81,* 945-960. (3)

Holm, K. (1983). Single subject research. *Nursing Research, 32,* 253-255. (5, 17)

Holm, R. A. (1981). Using data logging equipment. In E. E. Filsinger & R. A. Lewis (Eds.), *Assessing marriage: New behavioral approaches.* Baltimore, MD: University Park Press. (12)

Holtzclaw, B. J. (1990). Effects of extremity wraps to control drug-induced shivering: A pilot study. *Nursing Research, 39,* 280-283. (15)

House, J. S. (1981). *Work stress and social support.* Reading, MA: Addison-Wesley. (7)

Huang, H.-Y., Wilkie, D. J., & Berry, D. L. (1996). Use of a computerized digitizer tablet to score and enter visual analogue scale data. *Nursing Research, 45,* 370-372. (12)

Huang, Z., Hankinson, S. E., Colditz, G. A., Stampfer, M. J., Hunter, D. J., Manson, J. E., Hennekens, C. H., Rosner, B., Speizer, F. E., & Willett, W. C. (1997). Dual effects of weight and weight gain on breast cancer risk. *Journal of the American Medical Association, 278,* 1407-1449. (6)

Hubbard, P., Muhlenkamp, A. F., & Brown, N. (1984). The relationship between social support and self-care practices. *Nursing Research, 33,* 266-270. (7)

Hunter, J. E., & Schmidt, F. L. (1990). *Methods of meta-analysis: Correcting error and bias in research findings.* Newbury Park, CA: Sage. (14)

Hunter, J. E., Schmidt, F. L., & Jackson, G. B. (1982). *Meta-analysis: Cumulating research findings across studies.* Beverly Hills, CA: Sage. (14)

Hurley, P. M. (1983). Communication variables and voice analysis of marital conflict stress. *Nursing Research, 32,* 164-169. (10)

Irvine, D. M., & Evans, M. G. (1995). Job satisfaction and turnover among nurses: Integrating research findings across studies. *Nursing Research, 44,* 246-253. (14)

Jacobsen, B. S., & Meininger, J. C. (1986). Randomized experiments in nursing: The quality of reporting. *Nursing Research, 35,* 379-382. (5, 20)

Jacobsen, B. S., & Meininger, J. C. (1990). Seeing the importance of blindness. *Nursing Research, 39,* 54-57. (5)

Jacobsen, B. S., Tulman, L., & Lowery, B. J. (1991). Three sides of the same coin: The analysis of paired data from dyads. *Nursing Research, 40,* 359-363. (10)

Janke, J. R. (1994). Development of the breast-feeding attrition prediction tool. *Nursing Research, 43,* 100-104. (16)

Janken, J. K., Reynolds, B. A., & Swiech, K. (1986). Patient falls in the acute care setting: Identifying risk factors. *Nursing Research, 35,* 215-219. (8)

Johnson, J. E. (1966). The influence of a purposeful nurse-patient interaction on the patients' postoperative course. In *Exploring progress in medical-surgical nursing practice* (pp. 16-22). New York: American Nurses Association. (1)

Johnson, J. E. (1973). Effects of accurate expectations about sensations on the sensory and distress components of pain. *Journal of Personality and Social Psychology, 27,* 261-275. (1)

Johnson, J. E. (1996). Coping with radiation therapy: Optimism and the effect of preparatory interventions. *Research in Nursing & Health, 19,* 3-12. (1, 5)

Johnson, J. E., & Lauver, D. R. (1989). Alternative explanations of coping with stressful experiences associated with physical illness. *Advances in Nursing Science, 11*(2), 39-52. (1)

Johnson, J. L., Ratner, P. A., Bottorff, J. L., & Hayduk, L. A. (1993). An exploration of Pender's Health Promotion Model using LISREL. *Nursing Research, 42,* 132-138. (7, 11, 13)

Jones, E. (1987). Translation of quantitative measures for use in cross-cultural research. *Nursing Research, 36,* 324-327. (10)

Jones, E. G. (1995). Deaf and hearing parents' perceptions of family functioning. *Nursing Research, 44,* 102-105. (8)

Jones, K. R. (1992). Risk of hospitalization for chronic hemodialysis patients. *Image, 24,* 88-94. (11)

Julian, T. W., & Knapp, T. R. (1995). The National Survey of Families and Households: A rich database for nursing research. *Research in Nursing & Health, 18,* 173-177. (13)

Kawachi, I., Colditz, G. A., Speizer, F. E., Manson, J. E., Stampfer, M. J., Willett, W. C., & Hennekens, C. H. (1997). A prospective study of passive smoking and coronary heart disease. *Circulation, 95,* 2374-2379. (6)

Keefe, M. R., Kotzer, A. M., Froese-Fretz, A., & Curtin, M. (1996). A longitudinal comparison of irritable and nonirritable infants. *Nursing Research, 45,* 4-9. (8)

Keller, E., & Bzdek, V. M. (1986). Effects of therapeutic touch on tension headache pain. *Nursing Research, 35,* 101-106. (9)

Kiecolt, K. J., & Nathan, L. E. (1985). *Secondary analysis of survey data.* Beverly Hills, CA: Sage. (13)

Kiger, J., & Murphy, S. A. (1987). Reliability assessment of the SCL-90-R using a longitudinal bereaved disaster population. *Western Journal of Nursing Research, 9,* 572-588. (8)

Kimchi, J., Polivka, B., & Stevenson, J. S. (1991). Triangulation: Operational definitions. *Nursing Research, 40,* 364-366. (10)

King, K. B., Norsen, L. H., Robertson, K. R., & Hicks, G. L. (1987). Patient management of pain medication after cardiac surgery. *Nursing Research, 36,* 145-150. (9)

Kinney, M. R., Burfitt, S. N., Stullenbarger, E., Rees, B., & DeBolt, M. R. (1996). Quality of life in cardiac patient research. *Nursing Research, 45,* 173-180. (14)

Kirk, R. E. (1996). Practical significance: A concept whose time has come. *Educational and Psychological Measurement, 56,* 746-759. (11)

Knapp, T. R. (1985). Validity, reliability, and neither. *Nursing Research, 37,* 189-192. (10)

Knapp, T. R. (1988). Stress versus strain: A methodological critique. *Nursing Research, 37,* 181-184. (10)

Knapp, T. R. (1990). Treating ordinal scales as interval scales: An attempt to resolve the controversy. *Nursing Research, 39,* 121-123. (10, 16)

Knapp, T. R. (1991). Coefficient alpha: Conceptualizations and anomalies. *Research in Nursing & Health, 14,* 457-460. (10)

Knapp, T. R. (1993). Treating ordinal scales as ordinal scales. *Nursing Research, 42,* 184-186. (10, 16)

Knapp, T. R. (1994a). Regression analyses: What to report. *Nursing Research, 43,* 187-189. (11, 20)

Knapp, T. R. (1994b). Supply (of journal space) and demand (by assistant professors). *Image, 26,* 247. (20)

Knapp, T. R. (1996a). *Learning statistics through playing cards.* Thousand Oaks, CA: Sage. (11)

Knapp, T. R. (1996b). The overemphasis on power analysis. *Nursing Research, 45,* 379-381. (9)

Knapp, T. R. (1997). The prestige value of books and journal articles. *Nurse Educator, 22,* 10-11. (20)

Knapp, T. R., & Brown, J. K. (1995). Ten measurement commandments that often should be broken. *Research in Nursing & Health, 18,* 465-469. (10, 16)

Knapp, T. R., & Campbell-Heider, N. (1989). Numbers of observations and variables in multivariate analyses. *Western Journal of Nursing Research, 11,* 634-641. (9)

Knapp, T. R., Kimble, L. P., & Dunbar, S. B. (1998). Distinguishing between the stability of a construct and the stability of an instrument in trait/state measurement. *Nursing Research, 47,* 60-62. (10)

Kolanowski, A., Hurwitz, S., Taylor, L. A., Evans, L., & Strumpf, N. (1994). Contextual factors associated with disturbing behaviors in institutionalized elders. *Nursing Research, 43,* 73-79. (13)

Koniak-Griffin, D., & Brecht, M.-L. (1995). Linkages between sexual risk taking, substance abuse, and AIDS knowledge among pregnant adolescents and young mothers. *Nursing Research, 44,* 340-346. (7, 11)

Koniak-Griffin, S., & Ludington-Hoe, S. M. (1988). Developmental and temperament outcomes of sensory stimulation in healthy infants. *Nursing Research, 37,* 70-76. (10)

Kotch, J. B., Browne, D. C., Ringwalt, C. L., Stewart, W. P., Ruina, E., Holt, K., Lowman, B., & Jung, J. W. (1995). Risk of child abuse or neglect in a cohort of low-income children. *Child Abuse & Neglect, 19,* 1115-1130. (13)

Kovach, C. R., & Knapp, T. R. (1989). Age, cohort, and time-period confounds in research on aging. *Journal of Gerontological Nursing, 15*(3), 11-15. (8)

Kraemer, H. C., & Thiemann, S. (1987). *How many subjects?* Newbury Park, CA: Sage. (9)

Kraemer, H. C., & Thiemann, S. (1989). A strategy to use soft data effectively in randomized controlled clinical trials. *Journal of Consulting and Clinical Psychology, 57,* 148-154. (18, 19)

Krywanio, M. L. (1994). Meta-analysis of physiological outcomes of hospital-based infant intervention programs. *Nursing Research, 43,* 133-137. (14)

Kuhlman, G. J., Wilson, H. S., Hutchinson, S. A., & Wallhagen, M. (1991). Alzheimer's disease and family caregiving: Critical synthesis of the literature and research agenda. *Nursing Research, 40,* 331-337. (14)

Labyak, S. E., & Metzger, B. L. (1997). The effects of effleurage backrub on the physiological components of relaxation: A meta-analysis. *Nursing Research, 46,* 59-62. (14)

Lander, J., Nazarali, S., Hodgins, M., Friesen, E., McTavish, J., Ouellette, J., & Abel, R. (1996). Evaluation of a new topical anesthetic agent: A pilot study. *Nursing Research, 45,* 50-53. (15)

Landis, C. A., & Whitney, J. D. (1997). Effects of 72 hours sleep deprivation on wound healing in the rat. *Research in Nursing & Health, 20,* 259-267. (4, 5)

LaRocco, J. M., House, J. S., & French, J. R. (1980). Social support, occupational stress and health. *Journal of Health and Social Behavior, 21,* 202-218. (7)

Larson, E. (1986). Evaluating validity of screening tests. *Nursing Research, 35,* 186-188. (10)

Larson, J. L., Covey, M. K., Vitalo, C. A., Alex, C. G., Patel, M., & Kim, M. J. (1996). Reliability and validity of the 12-minute distance walk in patients with chronic obstructive pulmonary disease. *Nursing Research, 45,* 203-210. (10)

Lattavo, K., Britt, J., & Dobal, M. (1995). Agreement between measures of pulmonary artery and tympanic temperatures. *Research in Nursing & Health, 18,* 365-370. (10)

Lauver, D., Nabholz, S., Scott, K., & Tak, Y. (1997). Testing theoretical explanations of mammography use. *Nursing Research, 46,* 32-39. (11)

Lauver, D., & Tak, Y. (1995). Optimism and coping with a breast cancer symptom. *Nursing Research, 44,* 202-207. (2)

Leathers, C. W. (1990). Choosing the animal: Reasons, excuses, and welfare. In B. E. Rollin & M. L. Kesel (Eds.), *The experimental animal in biomedical research,* Vol. 1: *A survey of scientific and ethical issues for investigators* (pp. 67-79). Boca Raton, FL: CRC. (4)

Lee, K. A., & Kieckhefer, G. M. (1989). Measuring human responses using visual analogue scales. *Western Journal of Nursing Research, 11,* 128-132. (10)

LeFort, S. M. (1992). The statistical versus clinical significance debate. *Image, 25,* 57-62. (11)

Leidy, N. K., Abbott, R. D., & Fedenko, K. M. (1997). Sensitivity and reproducibility of the dual-mode actigraph under controlled levels of activity intensity. *Nursing Research, 46,* 5-11. (10)

Leidy, N. K., & Weissfeld, L. A. (1991). Sample sizes and power computation for clinical intervention trials. *Western Journal of Nursing Research, 13,* 138-144. (5)

Leveck, M. L., & Jones, C. B. (1996). The nursing practice environment, staff retention, and quality of care. *Research in Nursing & Health, 19,* 331-343. (11)

Levine, R. J. (1986). *Ethics and regulation of clinical research* (2nd ed.). Baltimore, MD: Urban & Schwarzenberg. (4)

Likert, R. (1932). A technique for the assessment of attitudes. *Archives of Psychology, 22,* 5-55. (10)

Lin, P.-E., & Stivers, L. E. (1974). On differences of means with incomplete data. *Biometrika, 61,* 325-334. (19)

Lindenberg, C. S., Alexander, E. M., Gendrop, S. C., Nencioli, M., & Williams, D. G. (1991). A review of the literature on cocaine abuse in pregnancy. *Nursing Research, 40,* 69-75. (14)

Lindley, P., & Walker, S. N. (1993). Theoretical and methodological differentiation of moderation and mediation. *Nursing Research, 42,* 276-279. (3)

Little, R. J. A., & Rubin, D. B. (1987). *Statistical analysis with missing data.* New York: John Wiley. (19)

Lobo, M. (1986). Secondary analysis as a strategy for nursing research. In P. L. Chinn (Ed.), *Nursing research methodology* (pp. 295-304). Rockville, MD: Aspen. (13)

Logsdon, M. C., McBride, A. B., & Birkimer, J. C. (1994). Social support and postpartum depression. *Research in Nursing & Health, 17,* 449-457. (11)

Long, K. A., & Boik, R. J. (1993). Predicting alcohol use in rural children: A longitudinal study. *Nursing Research, 42,* 79-86. (11)

Lowe, N. K., Walker, S. N., & MacCallum, R. C. (1991). Confirming the theoretical structure of the McGill Pain Questionnaire in acute clinical pain. *Pain, 46,* 53-60. (10)

Lowery, B. J., & Jacobsen, B. S. (1984). On the consequences of overturning turnover: A study of performance and turnover. *Nursing Research, 33,* 363-367. (8)

Lucas, M. D., Atwood, J. R., & Hagaman, R. (1993). Replication and validation of Anticipated Turnover Model for urban registered nurses. *Nursing Research, 42,* 29-35. (11, 15)

Lynn, M. R. (1986). Determination and quantification of content validity. *Nursing Research, 35,* 382-385. (10)

Lynn, M. R. (1989). Meta-analysis: Appropriate tool for the integration of nursing research? *Nursing Research, 38,* 302-305. (14)

Macnee, C. L., & Talsma, A. (1995). Development and testing of the Barriers to Cessation Scale. *Nursing Research, 44,* 214-219. (16)

Mahon, N. E., & Yarcheski, A. (1988). Loneliness in early adolescents: An empirical test of alternate explanations. *Nursing Research, 37,* 330-335. (15)

Mahon, N. E., & Yarcheski, A. (1992). Alternate explanations of loneliness in adolescents: A replication and extension study. *Nursing Research, 41,* 151-156. (15)

Mahon, N. E., Yarcheski, T. J., & Yarcheski, A. (1995). Validation of the Revised UCLA Loneliness Scale for adolescents. *Research in Nursing & Health, 18,* 263-270. (10)

Manson, J. E., Colditz, G. A., Stampfer, M. J., Willett, W. C., Rosner, B., Monson, R. R., Speizer, F. E., & Hennekens, C. H. (1990). A prospective study of obesity and risk of coronary heart disease in women. *New England Journal of Medicine, 322,* 882-889. (6)

Manson, J. E., Willett, W. C., Stampfer, M. J., Colditz, G. A., Hunter, D. J., Hankinson, S. E., Hennekens, C. H., & Speizer, F. E. (1995). Body weight and mortality among women. *New England Journal of Medicine, 333*, 677-685. (6)

Marascuilo, L. A., & Levin, J. R. (1983). *Multivariate statistics in the social sciences.* Pacific Grove, CA: Brooks/Cole. (11, 19)

Marcus-Roberts, H., & Roberts, F. (1987). Meaningless statistics. *Journal of Educational Statistics, 12,* 383-394. (10, 11)

Markowitz, J. S., Pearson, G., Kay, B. G., & Loewenstein, R. (1981). Nurses, physicians, and pharmacists: Their knowledge of hazards of medications. *Nursing Research, 30,* 366-370. (9)

Mason-Hawkes, J., & Holm, K. (1989). Causal modeling: A comparison of path analysis and LISREL. *Nursing Research, 38,* 312-314. (11)

Mayo, D. J., Horne, M. K., III, Summers, B. L., Pearson, D. C., & Helsabeck, C. B. (1996). The effects of heparin flush on patency of the Groshong catheter. *Oncology Nursing Forum, 23,* 1401-1405. (5, 11, 15)

McArt, E. W., & McDougal, L. W. (1985). Secondary analysis: A new approach to nursing research. *Image, 17,* 54-57. (13)

McCaffery, M., Ferrell, B. R., & Turner, M. (1996). Ethical issues in the use of placebos in cancer pain management. *Oncology Nursing Forum, 23,* 1587-1593. (4)

McDougall, G. J. (1994). Predictors of metamemory in older adults. *Nursing Research, 43,* 212-218. (8)

McGuire, D. (1984). The measurement of clinical pain. *Nursing Research, 33,* 152-156. (10)

McKeown, B., & Thomas, D. (1988). *Q methodology.* Newbury Park, CA: Sage. (10)

McLaughlin, F. E., & Marascuilo, L. A. (1990). *Advanced nursing and health care research: Quantification approaches.* Philadelphia: W. B. Saunders. (5, 11, 17)

McPhail, A., Pikula, H., Roberts, J., Browne, G., & Harper, D. (1990). Primary nursing: A randomized crossover trial. *Western Journal of Nursing Research, 12,* 188-200. (5)

Medoff-Cooper, B., & Brooten, D. (1987). Relation of the feeding cycle to neurobehavioral assessment in preterm infants: A pilot study. *Nursing Research, 36,* 315-317. (10, 15)

Medoff-Cooper, B., Delivoria-Papadopoulos, M., & Brooten, D. (1991). Serial neurobehavioral assessments of preterm infants. *Nursing Research, 40,* 94-97. (8)

Medoff-Cooper, B., & Gennaro, S. (1996). The correlation of sucking behaviors and Bayley Scales of Infant Development at six months of age in VLBW infants. *Nursing Research, 45,* 291-296. (2)

Melnyk, B. M., Alpert-Gillis, L. J., Hensel, P. B., Cable-Beiling, R. C., & Rubenstein, J. S. (1997). Helping mothers cope with a critically ill child: A pilot test of the COPE intervention. *Research in Nursing & Health, 20,* 3-14. (5, 15)

Menard, S. (1995). *Applied logistic regression analysis.* Thousand Oaks, CA: Sage. (11)

Mercer, R. T., & Ferketich, S. L. (1990a). Predictors of family functioning eight months following birth. *Nursing Research, 39,* 76-82. (8)

Mercer, R. T., & Ferketich, S. L. (1990b). Predictors of parental attachment during early parenthood. *Journal of Advanced Nursing, 15,* 268-280. (8)

Mercer, R. T., & Ferketich, S. L. (1993). Predictors of partner relationships during pregnancy and infancy. *Research in Nursing & Health, 16,* 45-56. (8)

Mercer, R. T., & Ferketich, S. L. (1994a). Maternal-infant attachment of experienced and inexperienced mothers during infancy. *Nursing Research, 43,* 344-351. (8)

Mercer, R. T., & Ferketich, S. L. (1994b). Predictors of maternal role competence by risk status. *Nursing Research, 43,* 38-43. (8)

Mercer, R. T., & Ferketich, S. L. (1995). Experienced and inexperienced mothers' maternal competence during infancy. *Research in Nursing & Health, 18,* 333-343. (8)

Mercer, R. T., Ferketich, S. L., DeJoseph, J., May, K. A., & Sollid, D. (1988). Effect of stress on family functioning during pregnancy. *Nursing Research, 37,* 268-275. (8)

Mercer, R. T., May, K. A., Ferketich, S., & DeJoseph, J. (1986). Theoretical models for studying the effects of antepartum stress on the family. *Nursing Research, 39,* 339-346. (8)

Milgram, S. (1974). *Obedience to authority: An experimental view.* New York: Harper & Row. (4)

Miller, A. M., & Champion, V. L. (1996). Mammography in older women: One-time and three-year adherence to guidelines. *Nursing Research, 45,* 239-245. (6, 9)

Miller, J. F., & Powers, M. J. (1988). Development of an instrument to measure hope. *Nursing Research, 37,* 6-10. (16)

Miller, L. L., Hornbrook, M. C., Archbold, P. G., & Stewart, B. J. (1996). Development of use and cost measures in a nursing intervention for family caregivers and frail elderly patients. *Research in Nursing & Health, 19,* 273-285. (5, 15)

Miller, P., Wikoff, R., Garrett, M. J., McMahon, M., & Smith, T. (1990). Regimen compliance two years after myocardial infarction. *Nursing Research, 39,* 333-336. (5)

Mills, E. M. (1994). The effect of low-intensity aerobic exercise on muscle strength, flexibility, and balance among sedentary elderly persons. *Nursing Research, 43,* 207-211. (5)

Mishel, M. H., Padilla, G., Grant, M., & Sorenson, D. S. (1991). Uncertainty in illness theory: A replication of the mediating effects of mastery and coping. *Nursing Research, 40,* 236-240. (15)

Mishel, M. H., & Sorenson, D. S. (1991). Uncertainty in gynecological cancer: A test of the mediating functions of mastery and coping. *Nursing Research, 40,* 167-171. (15)

Mitchell, E. S. (1986). Multiple triangulation: A methodology for nursing science. *Advances in Nursing Science, 8*(3), 18-26. (10)

Morgan, B. S. (1984). A semantic differential measure of attitudes toward black American patients. *Research in Nursing & Health, 7,* 155-162. (10)

Muchinsky, P. M. (1996). The correction for attenuation. *Educational and Psychological Measurement, 56,* 63-75. (10)

Munro, B. H. (1980). Dropouts from nursing education: Path analysis of a national sample. *Nursing Research, 29,* 371-377. (13)

Munro, B. H. (1983). Job satisfaction among recent graduates of schools of nursing. *Nursing Research, 32,* 350-355. (13)

Munro, B. H. (1985). Predicting success in graduate clinical specialty programs. *Nursing Research, 34,* 54-57. (7, 11)

Munro, B. H. (1997). *Statistics for health care research* (3rd ed.). Philadelphia: Lippincott. (10, 11, 12)

Munro, B. H., & Sexton, D. L. (1984). Path analysis: A method for theory testing. *Western Journal of Nursing Research, 6,* 97-106. (11)

Murdaugh, C. (1981). Measurement error and attenuation. *Western Journal of Nursing Research, 3,* 252-256. (10)

Murphy, S. A. (1984). Stress levels and health status of victims of a natural disaster. *Research in Nursing & Health, 7,* 205-215. (8)

Murphy, S. A. (1986a). Perceptions of stress, coping, and recovery one and three years after a natural disaster. *Issues in Mental Health Nursing, 8,* 63-77. (8)

Murphy, S. A. (1986b). Status of natural disaster victims' health and recovery three years later. *Research in Nursing & Health, 8,* 331-340. (8)

Murphy, S. A. (1987). Self-efficacy and social support: Mediators of stress on mental health following a natural disaster. *Western Journal of Nursing Research, 9,* 58-86. (8)

Murphy, S. A. (1988). Mental distress and recovery in a high-risk bereavement sample three years after untimely death. *Nursing Research, 37,* 30-35. (8, 9)

Murphy, S. A. (1989a). An explanatory model of recovery from disaster loss. *Research in Nursing & Health, 12,* 67-76. (8)

Murphy, S. A. (1989b). Multiple triangulation: Applications in a program of nursing research. *Nursing Research, 38,* 294-297. (8, 16)

Murphy, S. A., & Stewart, B. J. (1985-1986). Linked pairs of subjects: A method for increasing the sample size in a study of bereavement. *Omega, 16,* 141-153. (8, 9)

Nativio, D. G. (1993). Authorship. *Image, 25,* 358. (20)

Naylor, M. D. (1990). Comprehensive discharge planning for hospitalized elderly: A pilot study. *Nursing Research, 39,* 156-161. (15)

Neuberger, G. B., Kasal, S., Smith, K. V., Hassanein, R., & DeViney, S. (1994). Determinants of exercise and aerobic fitness in outpatients with arthritis. *Nursing Research, 43,* 11-17. (16)

Neuliep, J. W. (Ed.). (1991). *Replication research in the social sciences.* Newbury Park, CA: Sage. (15)

Nevo, B. (1985). Face validity revisited. *Journal of Educational Measurement, 22,* 287-293. (10)

Nield, M., & Gocka, I. (1993). To correlate or not to correlate: What is the question? *Nursing Research, 42,* 294-296. (10)

Norbeck, J. S. (1985). Types and sources of social support for managing job stress in critical care nursing. *Nursing Research, 34,* 225-230. (7)

Norbeck, J. S., Lindsey, A. M., & Carrieri, V. L. (1981). The development of an instrument to measure social support. *Nursing Research, 30,* 264-269. (10)

Norbeck, J. S., Lindsey, A. M., & Carrieri, V. L. (1983). Further development of the Norbeck Social Support Questionnaire: Normative data and validity testing. *Nursing Research, 32,* 4-9. (10)

Norman, E., Gadaleta, D., & Griffin, C. C. (1991). An evaluation of three blood pressure methods in a stabilized acute trauma population. *Nursing Research, 40,* 86-89. (1)

Northouse, L. L., Jeffs, M., Cracchiolo-Caraway, A., Lampman, L., & Dorris, G. (1995). Emotional distress reported by women and husbands prior to a breast biopsy. *Nursing Research, 44,* 196-201. (2, 19)

Northouse, L. L., Laten, D., & Reddy, P. (1995). Adjustment of women and their husbands to recurrent breast cancer. *Research in Nursing & Health, 18,* 515-524. (19)

Norwood, S. L. (1996). The Social Support Apgar: Instrument development and testing. *Research in Nursing & Health, 19,* 143-152. (16)

Nunnally, J. C., & Bernstein, I. H. (1994). *Psychometric theory* (3rd ed.). New York: McGraw-Hill. (9, 10)

Oberst, M. T. (1982). Clinical versus statistical significance. *Cancer Nursing, 5,* 475-476. (11)

O'Flynn, A. (1982). Meta-analysis. *Nursing Research, 31,* 314-316. (14)

Osgood, C., Suci, G., & Tannenbaum, P. (1957). *The measurement of meaning.* Urbana: University of Illinois Press. (10)

O'Sullivan, A. L., & Jacobsen, B. S. (1992). A randomized trial of a health care program for first-time adolescent mothers and their infants. *Nursing Research, 41,* 210-215. (5)

Ouellette, M. D., MacVicar, M. G., & Harlan, J. (1986). Relationship between percent body fat and menstrual patterns in athletes and nonathletes. *Nursing Research, 35,* 330-333. (8)

Padilla, G. V. (1984). Reliability and validity of the independent variable. *Western Journal of Nursing Research, 6,* 138-140. (10)

Palmer, M. H., German, P. S., & Ouslander, J. G. (1991). Risk factors for urinary incontinence one year after nursing home admission. *Research in Nursing & Health, 14,* 405-412. (11, 13)

Pender, N. J., & Pender, A. R. (1986). Attitudes, subjective norms, and intentions to engage in health behaviors. *Nursing Research, 35,* 15-18. (6)

Pender, N. J., Walker, S. N., Sechrist, K. R., & Frank-Stromborg, M. (1990). Predicting health-promoting lifestyles in the workplace. *Nursing Research, 39,* 326-332. (11)

Pletsch, P. K. (1991). Prevalence of smoking in Hispanic women of childbearing age. *Nursing Research, 40,* 103-106. (13)

Pohl, J. M., Boyd, C., Liang, J., & Given, C. W. (1995). Analysis of the impact of mother-daughter relationships on the commitment to caregiving. *Nursing Research, 44,* 68-75. (11)

Polit, D. F. (1996). *Data analysis and statistics for nursing research.* Stamford, CT: Appleton & Lange. (11)

Polit, D. F., & Hungler, B. P. (1995). *Nursing research: Principles and methods* (5th ed.). Philadelphia: Lippincott. (7, 10, 12)

Polivka, B. J., & Nickel, J. T. (1992). Case-control design: An appropriate strategy for nursing research. *Nursing Research, 41,* 250-253, 380. (8)

Pollow, R. L., Stoller, E. P., Forster, L. E., & Duniho, T. S. (1994). Drug combinations and potential for risk of adverse drug reaction among community-dwelling elderly. *Nursing Research, 43,* 44-49. (11)

Powers, B. A., & Knapp, T. R. (1995). *A dictionary of nursing theory and research* (2nd ed.). Thousand Oaks, CA: Sage. (preface)

Powers, M. J., & Jalowiec, A. (1987). Profile of the well-controlled, well-adjusted hypertensive patient. *Nursing Research, 36,* 106-110. (10)

Pranulis, M. F. (1996). Protecting rights of human subjects. *Western Journal of Nursing Research, 18,* 474-478. (4)

Pranulis, M. F. (1997). Nurses' roles in protecting human subjects. *Western Journal of Nursing Research, 19,* 130-136. (4)

Prescott, P. A., & Soeken, K. L. (1989). The potential uses of pilot work. *Nursing Research, 38,* 60-62. (15)

Pugh, L. C., & DeKeyser, F. G. (1995). Use of physiologic variables in nursing research. *Image, 27,* 273-276. (10)

Puntillo, K., & Weiss, S. J. (1994). Pain: Its mediators and associated morbidity in critically ill cardiovascular surgical patients. *Nursing Research, 43,* 31-36. (10)

Quinless, F. W., & Nelson, M. A. M. (1988). Development of a measure of learned helplessness. *Nursing Research, 37,* 11-15. (16)

Ratner, P. A., Bottorff, J. L., Johnson, J. L., & Hayduk, L. A. (1994). The interaction effects of gender within the Health Promotion Model. *Research in Nursing & Health, 17,* 341-350. (11)

Ratner, P. A., Bottorff, J. L., Johnson, J. L., & Hayduk, L. A. (1996). Using multiple indicators to test the dimensionality of concepts in the Health Promotion Model. *Research in Nursing & Health, 19,* 237-247. (11)

Reed, K. S. (1992). The effect of gestational age and pregnancy planning status on obstetrical nurses' perceptions of giving emotional care to women experiencing miscarriage. *Image, 24,* 107-110. (9)

Rice, V. H., Caldwell, M., Butler, S., & Robinson, J. (1986). Relaxation training and response to cardiac catheterization: A pilot study. *Nursing Research, 35,* 39-43. (15)

Rock, D. L., Green, K. E., Wise, B. K., & Rock, R. D. (1984). Social support and social network scales: A psychometric review. *Research in Nursing & Health, 7,* 325-332. (10)

Rogers, A. E., Caruso, C. C., & Aldrich, M. (1993). Reliability of sleep diaries for assessment of sleep/wake patterns. *Nursing Research, 42,* 368-371. (10)

Rollin, B. E. (1990). Ethics and research animals: Theory and practice. In B. E. Rollin & M. L. Kesel (Eds.), *The experimental animal in biomedical research,* Vol. 1: *A survey of scientific and ethical issues for investigators* (pp. 19-34). Boca Raton, FL: CRC. (4)

Roseman, C., & Booker, J. M. (1995). Workload and environmental factors in hospital medication errors. *Nursing Research, 44,* 226-230. (2)

Rudy, E. B., Estok, P. J., Kerr, M. E., & Menzel, L. (1994). Research incentives: Money versus gifts. *Nursing Research, 43,* 253-255. (4)

Ryan, N. M. (1983). The epidemiological method of building causal inference. *Advances in Nursing Science, 5*(2), 73-81. (8)

Ryan-Wenger, N. M. (1990). Development and psychometric properties of the Schoolagers' Coping Strategies Inventory. *Nursing Research, 39,* 344-349. (10)

Salmeron, J., Manson, J. E., Stampfer, M. J., Colditz, G. A., Wing, A. L., & Willett, W. C. (1997). Dietary fiber, glycemic load, and risk of non-insulin-dependent diabetes mellitus in women. *Journal of the American Medical Association, 277,* 472-477. (6)

Samarel, N., Fawcett, J., & Tulman, L. (1997). Effect of support groups with coaching on adaptation to early stage breast cancer. *Research in Nursing & Health, 20,* 15-26. (5)

Sanchez-Guerrero, J., Colditz, G. A., Karlson, E. W., Hunter, D. J., Speizer, F. E., & Liang, M. H. (1995). Silicone breast implants and the risk of connective-tissue diseases and symptoms. *New England Journal of Medicine, 332,* 1666-1670. (6)

Sapontzis, S. F. (1990). The case against invasive research with animals. In B. E. Rollin & M. L. Kesel (Eds.), *The experimental animal in biomedical research,* Vol. 1: *A survey of scientific and ethical issues for investigators* (pp. 3-17). Boca Raton, FL: CRC. (4)

Schilke, J. M., Johnson, G. O., Housh, T. J., & O'Dell, J. R. (1996). Effects of muscle-strength training on the functional status of patients with osteoarthritis of the knee joint. *Nursing Research, 45,* 68-72. (5)

Schlesselman, J. J. (1982). *Case-control studies.* New York: Oxford University Press. (8)

Schlotfeldt, R. M. (1987). Defining nursing: A historic controversy. *Nursing Research, 36,* 64-67. (1)

Schraeder, B. D. (1986). Developmental progress in very low birth weight infants during the first year of life. *Nursing Research, 35,* 237-242. (7, 11)

Schraeder, B. D., & Medoff-Cooper, B. (1983). Development and temperament in very low birth weight infants: The second year. *Nursing Research, 32,* 331-335. (10)

Schultz, S. (1989). The incipient paradigm shift in statistical computing. In I. L. Abraham, D. M. Nadzam, & J. J. Fitzpatrick (Eds.), *Statistics and quantitative methods in nursing: Issues and strategies for research and education* (pp. 30-36). Philadelphia: W. B. Saunders. (12)

Sechrist, K. R., Walker, S. N., & Pender, N. J. (1987). Development and psychometric evaluation of the Exercise Benefits Barrier Scale. *Research in Nursing & Health, 10,* 357-365. (16)

Secolsky, C. (1987). On the direct measurement of face validity: A comment on Nevo. *Journal of Educational Measurement, 24,* 82-83. (10)

Seddon, J. M., Willett, W. C., Speizer, F. E., & Hankinson, S. E. (1996). A prospective study of cigarette smoking and age-related macular deterioration in women. *Journal of the American Medical Association, 276,* 1141-1146. (6)

Shacham, S., & Daut, R. (1981). Anxiety or pain: What does the scale measure? *Journal of Consulting and Clinical Psychology, 49,* 468-469. (10)

Shamansky, S. L., Schilling, L. S., & Holbrook, T. L. (1985). Determining the market for nurse practitioner services: The New Haven experience. *Nursing Research, 34,* 242-247. (6)

Sidani, S., & Lynn, M. R. (1993). Examining amount and pattern of change: Comparing repeated measures ANOVA and individual regression analysis. *Nursing Research, 42,* 283-286. (18, 19)

Siegel, S., & Castellan, N. J. (1988). *Nonparametric statistics for the behavioral sciences* (2nd ed.). New York: McGraw-Hill. (11)

Simpson, S. H. (1989). Use of Q-sort methodology in cross-cultural nutrition and health research. *Nursing Research, 38,* 289-290. (10)

Simpson, T., Lee, E. R., & Cameron, C. (1996). Relationships among sleep dimensions and factors that impair sleep after cardiac surgery. *Research in Nursing & Health, 19,* 213-223. (10)

Skoner, M. M., Thompson, W. D., & Caron, V. A. (1994). Factors associated with risk of stress urinary incontinence in women. *Nursing Research, 43,* 301-306. (8)

Slakter, M. J., Wu, Y.-W. B., & Suzuki-Slakter, N. S. (1991). *, **, and ***: Statistical nonsense at the .00000 level. *Nursing Research, 40,* 248-249. (11)

Smith, D. W., & Shamansky, S. L. (1983). Determining the market for family nurse practitioner services: The Seattle experience. *Nursing Research, 32,* 301-305. (6)

Smith, L. W. (1988). Microcomputer-based bibliographic searching. *Nursing Research, 37,* 125-127. (12)

Smyth, K. A., & Yarandi, H. N. (1992). A path model of Type A and Type B responses to coping and stress in employed black women. *Nursing Research, 41,* 260-265. (11)

Sommers, M. S., Woods, S. L., & Courtade, M. A. (1993). Issues in methods and measurement of thermodilution cardiac output. *Nursing Research, 42,* 228-233. (10)

Spees, C. M. (1991). Knowledge of medical terminology among clients and families. *Image, 23,* 225-229. (10)

Spence Laschinger, H. K. (1992). Intraclass correlations as estimates of interrater reliability in nursing research. *Western Journal of Nursing Research, 14,* 246-251. (10)

Staggers, N., & Mills, M. E. (1994). Nurse-computer interaction: Staff performance outcomes. *Nursing Research, 43,* 144-150. (12)

Stampfer, M. J., Colditz, G. A., Willett, W. C., Manson, J. E., Rosner, B., Speizer, F. E., & Hennekens, C. H. (1991). Postmenopausal estrogen therapy and cardiovascular disease. *New England Journal of Medicine, 325,* 756-762. (6)

Stampfer, M. J., Willett, W. C., Speizer, F. E., Dysert, D. C., Lipnick, R., Rosner, B., & Hennekens, C. H. (1984). Test of the National Death Index. *American Journal of Epidemiology, 119,* 837-839. (6)

Stephenson, W. (1953). *The study of behavior: Q-technique and its methodology.* Chicago: University of Chicago Press. (10)

Stevens, S. S. (1946). On the theory of scales of measurement. *Science, 103,* 677-680. (10)

Stewart, D. W., & Kamins, M. A. (1993). *Secondary research: Information sources and methods* (2nd ed.). Newbury Park, CA: Sage. (13)

Stokes, S. A., & Gordon, S. E. (1988). Development of an instrument to measure stress in the older adult. *Nursing Research, 37,* 16-19. (10, 16)

Strickland, O. L., & Waltz, C. F. (1986). Measurement of research variables in nursing. In P. L. Chinn (Ed.), *Nursing research methodology* (pp. 79-90). Rockville, MD: Aspen. (10)

Stuart, A. (1984). *The ideas of sampling* (3rd ed.). London: Griffin. (9)

Suter, W. N., Wilson, D., & Naqvi, A. (1991). Using slopes to measure directional change. *Nursing Research, 40,* 250-252. (18, 19)

Swanson, E. A., & McCloskey, J. C. (1982). The manuscript review process. *Image, 14,* 72-76. (20)

Swanson, E. A., McCloskey, J. C., & Bodensteiner, A. (1991). Publishing opportunities for nurses: A comparison of 92 U.S. journals. *Image, 23,* 33-38. (20)

Tabachnick, B. G., & Fidell, L. S. (1996). *Using multivariate statistics* (3rd ed.). New York: HarperCollins. (11, 19)

Tatsuoka, M. M. (1993). Elements of the general linear model. In G. Keren & C. Lewis (Eds.), *A handbook for data analysis in the behavioral sciences: Statistical issues* (pp. 3-41). Hillsdale, NJ: Lawrence Erlbaum. (11)

Tesler, M. D., Savedra, M. C., Holzemer, W. L., Wilkie, D. J., Ward, J. A., & Paul, S. M. (1991). The word-graphic rating scale as a measure of children's and adolescents' pain intensity. *Research in Nursing & Health, 14,* 361-371. (10)

Thomas, K. A. (1991). The emergence of body temperature biorhythm in preterm infants. *Nursing Research, 40,* 98-102. (17)

Thomas, S. D., Hathaway, D. K., & Arheart, K. L. (1992). Face validity. *Western Journal of Nursing Research, 14,* 109-112. (10)

Thomas, S. P., & Groer, M. W. (1986). Relationships of demographic, life-style, and stress variables to blood pressure in adolescents. *Nursing Research, 35,* 169-172. (7)

Thomson, P. C. (1995). A hybrid paired and unpaired analysis for the comparison of proportions. *Statistics in Medicine, 14,* 1463-1470. (19)

Tilden, V. P., Nelson, C. A., & May, B. A. (1990). Use of qualitative methods to enhance content validity. *Nursing Research, 39,* 172-175. (10)

Tilden, V. P., & Stewart, B. J. (1985). Problems in measuring reciprocity with difference scores. *Western Journal of Nursing Research, 7,* 381-385. (18)

Timmerman, G. M. (1996). The art of advertising for research subjects. *Nursing Research, 45,* 339-340, 344. (17)

Topf, M. (1986a). Response sets in questionnaire research. *Nursing Research, 35,* 119-121. (6, 10)

Topf, M. (1986b). Three estimates of interrater reliability for nominal data. *Nursing Research, 35,* 253-255. (10)

Topf, M. (1990). Increasing the validity of research results with a blend of laboratory and clinical strategies. *Image, 22,* 121-123. (5)

Trinkoff, A. M., Eaton, W. W., & Anthony, J. C. (1991). The prevalence of substance abuse among registered nurses. *Nursing Research, 40,* 172-175. (6, 8)

Tukey, J. W. (1977). *Exploratory data analysis.* Reading, MA: Addison-Wesley. (11)

Tulman, L., & Fawcett, J. (1996a). Biobehavioral correlates of functional status following diagnosis of breast cancer: Report of a pilot study. *Image, 28,* 181. (15)

Tulman, L., & Fawcett, J. (1996b). Lessons learned from a pilot study of biobehavioral correlates of functional status in women with breast cancer. *Nursing Research, 45,* 356-358. (15)

Tyzenhouse, P. S. (1981). The nursing clinical trial. *Western Journal of Nursing Research, 3,* 102-109. (5)

Ventura, J. N. (1982). Parent coping behaviors, parent functioning and infant temperament characteristics. *Nursing Research, 31,* 268-273. (15)

Ventura, J. N. (1986). Parent coping: A replication. *Nursing Research, 35,* 77-80. (15)

Ventura, M. R., Hageman, P. T., Slakter, M. J., & Fox, R. N. (1980). Interrater reliabilities for two measures of nursing care quality. *Research in Nursing & Health, 3,* 25-32. (10)

Verran, J., & Ferketich, S. L. (1987a). Exploratory data analysis: Comparison of groups and variables. *Western Journal of Nursing Research, 9,* 617-625. (11)

Verran, J., & Ferketich, S. L. (1987b). Exploratory data analysis: Examining single distributions. *Western Journal of Nursing Research, 9,* 142-149. (11)

Voda, A. M., Inle, M., & Atwood, J. R. (1980). Quantification of self-report data from two-dimensional body diagrams. *Western Journal of Nursing Research, 2,* 707-729. (10)

Vortherms, R., Ryan, P., & Ward, S. (1992). Knowledge of, attitudes toward, and barriers to pharmacologic management of cancer pain in a statewide random sample of nurses. *Research in Nursing & Health, 15,* 459-466. (9)

Wagner, T. J. (1985). Smoking behavior of nurses in western New York. *Nursing Research, 34,* 58-60. (6, 9, 16)

Walker, S. N., Kerr, M. J., Pender, N. J., & Sechrist, K. R. (1990). A Spanish language version of the Health-Promoting Lifestyle Profile. *Nursing Research, 39,* 268-273. (10)

Waltz, C. F., Strickland, O. L., & Lenz, E. R. (1991). *Measurement in nursing research* (2nd ed.). Philadelphia: Davis. (10)

Wambach, K. A. (1997). Breastfeeding intention and outcome: A test of the theory of planned behavior. *Research in Nursing & Health, 20,* 51-59. (11)

Weaver, T. E., & Narsavage, G. L. (1992). Physiological and psychological variables related to functional status in chronic obstructive lung disease. *Nursing Research, 41,* 286-291. (11, 13)

Weaver, T. E., Richmond, T. S., & Narsavage, G. L. (1997). An explanatory model of functional status in chronic obstructive pulmonary disease. *Nursing Research, 46,* 26-31. (11, 13)

Webb, E. J., Campbell, D. T., Schwartz, R. B., Sechrest, L., & Grove, J. B. (1981). *Nonreactive measures in the social sciences* (2nd ed.). Boston: Houghton Mifflin. (10)

Weekes, D. P., & Rankin, S. H. (1988). Life-span developmental methods: Application to nursing research. *Nursing Research, 37,* 380-383. (8)

Weinert, C., & Tilden, V. P. (1990). Measures of social support. *Nursing Research, 39,* 212-216. (10)

Weiss, S. J. (1992). Measurement of the sensory qualities in tactile interaction. *Nursing Research, 41,* 82-86. (10)

Westfall, L. E. (1993). Animals, care, and nursing research. *Western Journal of Nursing Research, 15,* 568-581. (4)

Wewers, M. E., & Lowe, N. K. (1990). A critical review of visual analogue scales in the measurement of clinical phenomena. *Research in Nursing & Health, 13,* 227-236. (10)

White, M. A., & Wear, E. (1980). Parent-child separation: An observational methodology. *Western Journal of Nursing Research, 2,* 758-760. (12)

White, M. A., Wear, E., & Stephenson, G. (1983). A computer-compatible method for observing falling asleep behavior of hospitalized children. *Research in Nursing & Health, 6,* 191-198. (12)

Wikblad, K., & Anderson, B. (1995). A comparison of three wound dressings in patients undergoing heart surgery. *Nursing Research, 44,* 312-316. (5)

Wilkie, D. J., Savedra, M. C., Holzemer, W. L., Tesler, M. D., & Paul, S. M. (1990). Use of the McGill Pain Questionnaire to measure pain: A meta-analysis. *Nursing Research, 39,* 36-41. (14)

Willett, W. C., Browne, M. L., Bain, C., Lipnick, R. J., Stampfer, M. J., Rosner, B., Colditz, G. A., & Hennekens, C. H. (1985). Relative weight and risk of breast cancer among premenopausal women. *American Journal of Epidemiology, 122,* 731-740. (6)

Willett, W. C., Manson, J. E., Stampfer, M. J., Colditz, G. A., Rosner, B., Speizer, F. E., & Hennekens, C. H. (1995). Weight, weight change, and coronary heart disease in women. *Journal of the American Medical Association, 273,* 461-465. (6)

Willett, W. C., Stampfer, M. J., Manson, J. E., Colditz, G. A., Rosner, B. A., Speizer, F. E., & Hennekens, C. H. (1996). Coffee consumption and coronary heart disease in women. *Journal of the American Medical Association, 275,* 458-462. (6)

Williams, R. L., Thomas, S. P., Young, D. O., Jozwiak, J. J., & Hector, M. A. (1991). Development of a health habits scale. *Research in Nursing & Health, 14,* 145-153. (16)

Williamson, J. D., Karp, D. A., Dalphin, J. R., & Gray, P. S. (1982). *The research craft* (2nd ed.). Boston: Little, Brown. (3)

Wineman, N. M. (1990). Adaptation to multiple sclerosis: The role of social support, functional disability, and perceived uncertainty. *Nursing Research, 39,* 294-299. (11)

Wineman, N. M., & Durand, E. (1992). Incentives and rewards for subjects in nursing research. *Western Journal of Nursing Research, 14,* 526-531. (4)

Wineman, N. M., Durand, E. J., & McCulloch, B. J. (1994). Examination of the factor structure of the Ways of Coping Questionnaire with clinical populations. *Nursing Research, 43,* 268-273. (10, 19)

Wineman, N. M., Durand, E. J., & Steiner, R. P. (1994). A comparative analysis of coping behaviors in persons with multiple sclerosis or a spinal cord injury. *Research in Nursing & Health, 17,* 185-194. (8)

Winslow, B. W. (1997). Effects of formal supports on stress outcomes in family caregivers of Alzheimer's patients. *Research in Nursing & Health, 20,* 27-37. (11)

Wolf, F. M. (1986). *Meta-analysis.* Beverly Hills, CA: Sage. (14)

Woolley, A. S. (1984). Questioning the mailed questionnaire as a valid instrument for research in nursing education. *Image, 16,* 115-119. (6, 10)

World Health Organization. (1977). *Manual of the international statistical classification of diseases, injuries, and causes of death.* Geneva: Author. (3)

Wu, Y.-W. B. (1995). Hierarchical linear models: A multilevel data analysis technique. *Nursing Research, 44,* 123-126. (13, 16)

Wu, Y.-W. B., & Slakter, M. J. (1989). Analysis of covariance in nursing research. *Nursing Research, 38,* 306-308. (5, 18)

Yarandi, H. N. (1993). Coding dummy variables and calculating the relative risk in a logistic regression. *Nursing Research, 42,* 312-314. (12)

Yarandi, H. N., & Simpson, S. H. (1991). The logistic regression model and the odds of testing HIV positive. *Nursing Research, 40,* 372-373. (11)

Yarbro, C. H. (1995). Duplicate publication: Guidelines for nurse authors and editors. *Image, 27,* 57. (20)

Yarcheski, A., Mahon, N. E., & Yarcheski, T. J. (1997). Alternate models of positive health practices in adolescents. *Nursing Research, 46,* 85-92. (11)

Yarcheski, A., Scoloveno, M. A., & Mahon, N. E. (1994). Social support and well-being in adolescents: The mediating role of hopefulness. *Nursing Research, 43,* 288-292. (3, 7, 11)

Yates, M. A. (1985). Cost savings as an indicator of successful nursing intervention. *Nursing Research, 34,* 50-53. (5)

Youngblot, J. M., & Casper, G. R. (1993). Single-item indicators in nursing research. *Research in Nursing & Health, 16,* 459-465. (10)

Ziemer, M. M., Cooper, D. M., & Pigeon, J. G. (1995). Evaluation of a dressing to reduce nipple pain and improve nipple skin condition in breast-feeding women. *Nursing Research, 44,* 347-351. (5)

Zimmerman, L., & Yeaworth, R. (1986). Factors influencing career success in nursing. *Research in Nursing & Health, 9,* 179-185. (9, 16)

Index